Lose Weight With Live Foods

A 10 Week Plan to Lose Fat and Gain Health and Fitness Eating Live, Raw Foods

by Lani Rossetta, B.A., B.S.

Printed in Medford, OR
USA
Publisher: Leihuna Enterprises

ISBN # 0-9709866-7-X

Photos by Lani and Stan Rossetta
Art work by Lani Rossetta

Some of the recipes in this book are taken from the book, "We Love Your Body", copyright 1980, written by Lani Miller (Rossetta) and Diane (Chelsea) Rodgers. Most of the recipes were created by me through experimentation, creative combining, and tweaking other recipes with my own unique contribution according to my own tastes, preferences and availability of ingredients. I have come to appreciate simplicity in preparation of live foods--in time spent, number of ingredients and cost. It really is very easy to eat as nature intended. The real key is to eat a colorful variety of plant foods.

Disclaimer: This is not a nutrition book, written by a traditional dietitian. However, there is ample evidence of the value of eating one's food uncooked in the variety that the trees and plants of our planet provide. It is up to the reader to see his physician before beginning an eating plan such as this, especially if one has any serious health condition or concern. The author claims no responsibility for the reader's health or any difficulties that may arise from eating this food. All statements herein are from the author's personal experience or from research she has read in other books by experts in their field. Furthermore, this book makes no claims to cure any condition, and makes no diagnoses. That is up to your own personal doctor.

12 Benefits to Eating Live Foods

1. When we leave home on a trip, I don't have to worry, when we're three hours away, whether or not I've left the oven on.

2. The stovetop gives me an extra counter for my salad spinner and colander to drain.

3. The oven is a great place for soaking nuts, seeds and grains overnight, until they begin to sprout. They like a dark, warm (from pilot light) place to germinate.

4. I only have to shop one aisle in the supermarket---the produce aisle. In one store I shop I can get organic produce, dried fruit, raw nuts and grains from the bins, organic herbs and staples, such as olive oil, tamari sauce, sea vegetables and raw nut butters, all in one long aisle.

5. Dishes are easy to rinse. There's no solid grease, no bones, fat or meat pieces to separate out from the vegetable/fruit compost pile. Plus, the leftovers smell sweet and fresh.

6. Most fruit and many vegetables can sit in a bowl on the counter until ripened just right for eating.

7. I never have to read labels. This is real freedom. The natural packaging of organic fruits and vegetables don't require labels. All fats, protein, fiber, carbohydrates and calories are combined by Mother Nature in just the right proportions for each individual fruit, nut or vegetable.

8. I don't need to concern myself with whether there are cheap fillers like salt or sugar added to my produce choices, nor whether the fruits or veggies are enhanced with artificial colors or flavorings.

9. I never have to go into junk food or chain fast-food restaurants again. Temptation is rarely around me, and the few times I've been surrounded by good, cooked food, I don't feel deprived or tempted.

10. The "transformed" me feels so good about the way I look, the weight I've shed, the clothes I can fit into and my increased health and energy, that I will continue this eating plan as a lifestyle or way of life as long as I am able.

11. My tastebuds and olfactory lobes are so acute and sharp that I have learned to discern subtle taste differences and smells in different types of tomatoes, bananas, avocados, or nuts. I've become a raw foods gourmet.

12. And finally, fruits, nuts, vegetables, seeds, and especially sprouts are lively and kind of fun to hang around with. I paint my plate with a palette of assorted colors, flavors, textures and shapes naturally found in unprocessed and raw foods. I create a beautiful salad bowl or fruit mandala. I sit down, give gratitude and enjoy my meals in peace and beauty, sometimes accompanied by my favorite music. Other times I sit in the center of my outdoor labyrinth or on the porch glider. Life is good. It really is about the simple things. Especially, simplifying the food we eat and being able to turn back the clock and reap the many health-giving benefits.

LOSE WEIGHT WITH LIVE FOODS!

(A 10 WEEK PLAN TO LOSE FAT AND GAIN HEALTH AND FITNESS)

	Page #
Dedication	iii
Acknowledgements	iv
Preface	vi
Introduction	viii
Chapter I - Why Live Foods? And Other Questions	11
Chapter II - Ready, Get Set, Go!	21
a. Basic Equipment	
b. Re-Filling Your Refrigerator	
c. Preparing Your Pantry	
Chapter III - Drink to Your Health (Juices, Smoothies, Shakes, Milks)	35
Chapter IV - Lively Sprouts! Seeds, Nuts, Beans, Grains (Breads, Crackers, Cereals)	51
Chapter V - Snacks (Sweet, Spicy, Frozen, On-the-Go)	65
Chapter VI - Food Processor Magic (Sauces, Dips-Spreads, Butters, Salsas, Yogurts, Seed Cheeses)	75
Chapter VII - Versatile Veggies/Fabulous Fruits (Salads, Dressings, Pickled Veggies, Sea Vegetables, Soups, Condiments)	91
Chapter VIII - It's the Main Thing (Patties, Loaves, Main Dishes)	117
Chapter IX - Sweet Satisfactions (Balls, Cookies/Energy Bars, Cake, Frozen Delights)	123
Chapter X - Ten Weeks of Live Food Menus	133
Chapter XI - What's Next? After Ten Weeks and a Significant Weight Loss	151
Raw Food Websites	158
Recommended Reading	159
About the Author	160
Photos - Before and After	161
Recipe Index	163

DEDICATION

"Lose Weight With Live Foods!" is dedicated, as are most of my books, to my eight beautiful and healthy grandchildren. They are a joy. They are joyful. They are the children of the future. I enjoy every moment I spend with them. They keep me young more than anything except raw, living foods. Living foods will keep me young enough to play with them until they are grown. Thank you, Devri (a new vegetarian), Andrew, Benjamin, Rebekah, Aubrey, Jacob, Nicole, and Karli (our salad girl). (listed in order of age, from oldest to youngest)

I also dedicate this book to my four children, Heidi, Dan, Wendy and Christopher, the first three who have blessed their lives along with mine by having these children. (Christopher is not yet married.) I want to thank my husband, Stan, who is there for me for every project, idea, and endeavor I explore in my life. He is right beside me, assisting, supporting, contributing, and providing the expertise to help me construct any project or creation I might dream up. He gives me practical and honest feedback. If he doesn't like a new dish I enthusiastically created, he will tell me. Thank you, honey, for honesty. Though not a raw foodist, he eats whatever salad, sauce or sweet I prepare and has increased his raw fruit and vegetable intake 100%.

Finally, I dedicate this book to a most special person, my mother, Harriet, who was my role model as I grew up, who loved unconditionally and gave of herself unselfishly, as she raised four children. Today, at the age of 86, as mentally alert as you or I, she recently had a book of children's stories published, along with a friend, Peggy, who also contributed stories she had written for children. Their first book signing in a local book store was a wonderful success. The name of their book is "Grannies' Shorts". My hats go off to you, mom. You have written more stories and poems than I could ever imagine. You go, girl!

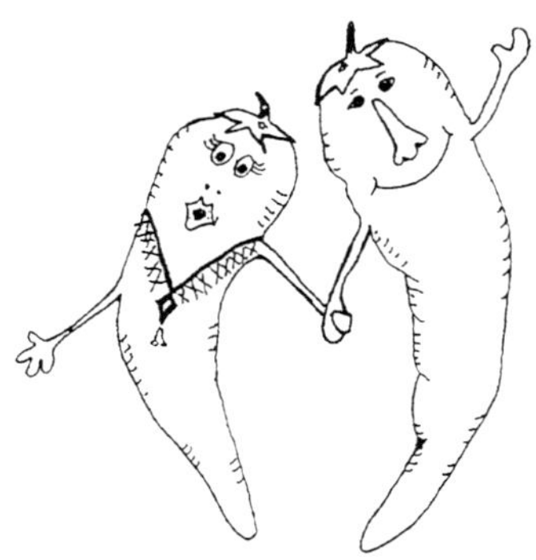

ACKNOWLEDGEMENTS

Thanks, first and foremost to the members of my first raw foods preparation class. Their feedback and the lessons I learned from that class have inspired some changes and new directions for my future classes. There were four women. I had them work in pairs, gave them each a menu with the recipes for preparing an entire luncheon. Between each recipe, once prepared and refrigerated, we went out to my garden labyrinth and did some standing yoga poses and deep breathing. That made a nice break. The food was tasty, according to everybody; sweet red pepper was omitted from one batch of sauce while three of the women, who get reflux sometimes, wish we had omitted the raw garlic from same sauce. I think we had too big of a selection of food items, because the salad alone had over 14 ingredients (lettuces, sprouts, etc.). There were too many different selections all in one meal. We were all stuffed. But the presentation was beautiful and colorful and they all enjoyed making it and tasting it all. There was plenty to take home to family. So, thank you, Cheryl, Bonny, Barb and Janet for helping me launch my new passion.

Thanks to my printer who works so closely with me during the publishing of my books. I do get a bit impatient sometimes, but the results are always exactly as I, the publisher, and author, want.

Thanks to the authors of the many raw foods books out there who so generously tell their own personal stories about their journey into raw foods and how they have benefited, as well as testimonials from their friends and students, declaring similar benefits. They taught me so much. I devoured each book, cover to cover, then set on my own journey to well-being-physically, mentally and spiritually. Losing weight was a goal, but really just an added benefit, compared to what I have reaped through the freedom I now have. I am no longer a slave to my taste buds and habits, nor to my supplements and looking at every new product on the market that I thought might help prevent this or cure that. I am free from all of that. I am feeling healthier and more fit each day. I feel in control of my health and not at the mercy of the latest research or warning or discovery. This is possible for you, too, just by changing your diet to raw and live foods. We *are* what we eat. I am at peace inside and feel so blessed to have had the right books and friends come into my life at just the right time.

Thanks to Shannon and Mike, living proof that one can have a busy life, family, and still eat raw. Thanks to the Boutenko family for their inspiring book, “Raw Family”. Both came into my life at exactly the right time. There are no accidents or plain coincidences in life. This was true synchronicity, displaying itself again in my life. Always there are synchronicities.

Last, but not least, a big thank you radiates out to my family. First, for the times I locked myself up in my kitchen, trying out new combinations, perfecting a recipe or asking them to try a new raw patty or sprouted bread. Thanks for understanding when I couldn't be with you or attend a basketball game or gymnastics meet because I spent a lot of time at my computer typing up the recipes to form this 10 week eating plan on live foods. Second, thanks for listening, and showing an interest in my latest, but very permanent enthusiasm for how I lost 25 pounds in 10 weeks. By your asking questions of me, then deciding to add more fruit and salads to your own diet and by tolerating my (hopefully) gentle nudges of encouragement to try more "raw", I feel I have solidified my own knowledge base and desire to benefit from the health and nutritional values of adding more live foods to my diet.

At the time of this writing my granddaughter phoned and announced that her dad (my oldest son) was out shopping for fruits and vegetables. They had decided as a family to try to eat more raw and live foods. My son, I knew, was interested, due to a persistent reflux-type disorder he has tolerated for several years, with no permanent relief. After hearing about live foods, he was considering trying it out. Now, it looks like they will try it as a family. What a way to provide support for each other and experiment with new fruits and taste sensations. It will be exciting, initially. I am positive the children can learn to add more raw fruits, veggies and nuts to their daily eating routine. Only time will tell how successful it is. I think it will be an interesting venture and I will surely be there for support and assistance if they need it. Email me if you are interested and I'll let you know the results.

I have *experienced* several months of eating live foods. I have *experienced* the feeling of well-being and increased health. Though I went 100% raw immediately, cold turkey, I can't expect that from less enthusiastic or less motivated friends and family. However, everyone travels their own journey at their own time and pace. As was once written, the journey of a 1000 miles begins with a single step. Let us all take that single step forward towards better health and fitness for a healthier body and planet.

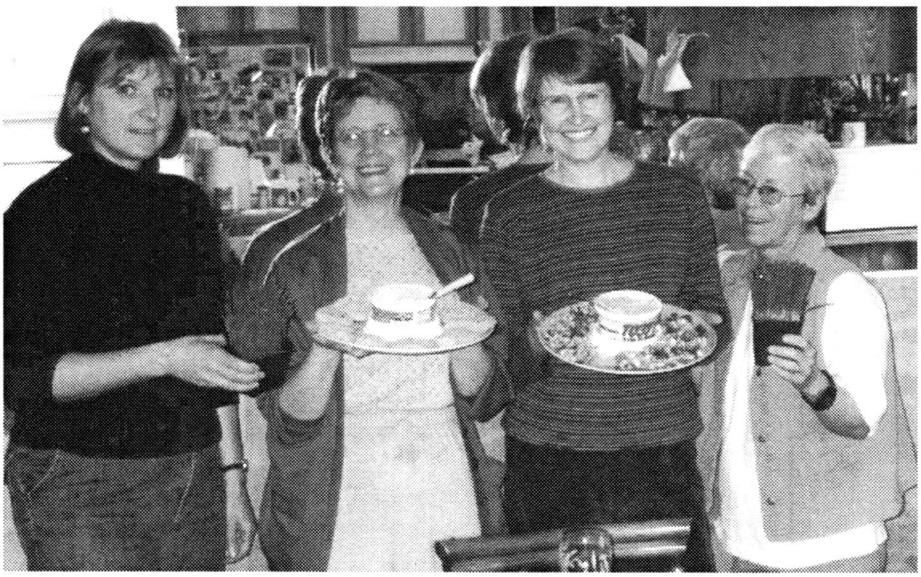

PREFACE

My first adventure into the raw food life occurred in 1980 when I was first becoming a vegetarian. My friend and business partner and I were running a natural foods snack bar at a local YMCA. Upon requests from our clients, we took a year to write down our recipes, creating a 256 page, vegetarian, natural nutrition and cookbook, "We Love Your Body". We incorporated living sprouts, lots of fresh fruit and salads into our book. However, we probably over-used honey, cheese and raw milk. We were both raising seven children between us and our book was written for parents who wanted to get their children off of junk food and into healthier eating. So our book was written as a transition book to healthy, vegetarian food. (At the time we thought unpasteurized honey from a local beekeeper, organic eggs, local cheese and raw milk from a friend's cow were the greatest discoveries since "ice cream".)

Well, we were on the right track. We made our own yogurt, sprouted our own seeds. I grew buckwheat lettuce, sunflower greens and wheat grass for juicing. I made tofu from scratch and tempeh with a culture I got from the agricultural department. I read "Survival into the 21st Century" by Viktoras Kulvinskas, a long time raw foodist, and incorporated some of his philosophy into my own, but I wasn't even close to thinking I (and my entire family) could eat raw and living foods, 100%.

Over the years I bought the juicing books and sprouting books. I met Ann Wigmore, in person, who is the queen of raw foods with her own personal healing story and the Hippocrates Health Institute that helps so many people improve their health through sprouts, wheat grass juice and raw, living foods. I would say, most definitively, that during the late 70's and early 80's the *seed* was planted. It just needed to incubate for another several years. And now, in 2003, I can say that the time was right. I needed to lose weight. I'd tried many "diets", including macrobiotics. Nothing worked for me. I had slowly gained 40 pounds from my normal weight of 115 pounds.

I look back now, and wonder why I didn't consider live foods. I think I just wanted to continue with my favorite "healthy" foods, as well as 'junk foods', just by cutting down the amounts. However, you know that if you have acquired habits and cravings for certain foods, it is very difficult to just cut down. For me I wanted to abstain, but my cravings got the best of me. They controlled *me!* Not only my cravings (both physical, or so I thought, and psychological) but my tastebuds controlled me, dictated to *me* what I would put in my mouth. I couldn't cut from three mochas to one mocha a week.

What use was it to eat really 'healthy' foods like beans and rice, steamed veggies or stir-fried veggies, whole wheat bread and decaffeinated mochas, if I also added pastas, a few candy bars, popcorn, and the inability to turn down sweets if they presented themselves to me in a social setting? I never bought cookies, crackers, pastries or pies, but watch out for the cakes and cookies if I was around--in the schools, at a meeting, at friends, or during a workshop.

Even cutting calories and some foods from my diet could not stave the cravings, nor release any pounds of fat. I thought my set point was my high weight and there was nothing I could do to lose even one pound. I exercised, so I was sure my metabolism wasn't too sluggish. This was very discouraging to me. So you can see what led up to this desire, when I had another birthday, to stop this craziness and get out of my rut by trying something completely (not really) different. My health appeared to be good, but there were several small concerns that might be leading me down the road to visit a doctor. I wanted better health, more energy and less "aging" concerns like stiff joints in the morning and a bum knee, among other things.

I was definitely sick of my "fat" wardrobe. I had kept most of my thin clothes, it being only 11 years since I was at my optimum weight. I figured I'd lose that 5 pounds, then 10 pounds, 20, 30 and finally 40. It wasn't about to happen all by itself. My personal desire couldn't make it happen. I had to decide that a great desire for better health and fitness, plus some action of a different kind, was the path to my destination or goal. Remaining status quo was no longer an option. And as it is known, when you put a desire out to the Universe, a burning desire, it always responds. Hence, the series of synchronous events that led me down this wonderful and exciting path to wellness. I hope you enjoy and can take with you even a few ideas to incorporate into your lifestyle that will lead you down your own path to health, fitness and freedom from excess 'fat'. I offer it to you in all sincerity and belief that it could work for you.

Namasté,

Lani Adair Bergquist Rossetta

Lani Adair Bergquist Rossetta

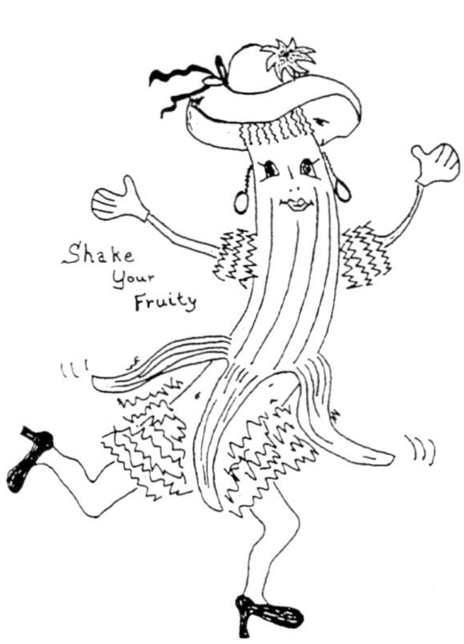

INTRODUCTION

In "Lose Weight With Live Foods" I am offering a ten-week plan to attain a healthier lifestyle, to feel great, enjoy having more energy than you are accustomed to, and, as a bonus, lose weight.

In this ten-week eating plan you will eliminate from your plate any processed or refined food, simple carbohydrates or foods with a high glycemic index, like potatoes, rice and breads. In other words, if it doesn't come directly from a plant, tree, bush or soil, you probably won't be consuming it.

The only fats you will be eating, other than that naturally present in fruits and vegetables (yes, there is a little fat in fruits and vegetables-especially seeds, nuts, olives and avocados), will be olive oil and flax oil.

All of your food will be raw and live. All fruit is fresh and uncooked or naturally dried without any preservatives. All vegetables are raw, not steamed or baked.

What seemed to me to be a difficult venture to undertake, especially 100%, turned out to be easier than if I had retained some cooked food in my diet. But that's just how I am. I couldn't see myself eating a baked potato or yam, cooked lentils and then something raw. I was sure the cooked foods would crowd out the raw and I'd go overboard again with starches, fats and sweets. My mochas, occasional candy bar and toast might over-shadow the benefits I'd be getting from the few fruits and vegetable salads I might add to my diet. By committing to eating 100% raw, I felt the battle was halfway won. Here are the benefits I noticed almost immediately:

1. I was rarely hungry. I could eat as many nuts, seeds, fruits, vegetables or sprouts as I wanted until I felt full.
2. I began to appreciate herbs and spices to flavor foods as well as the natural flavors of each individual fruit or vegetable.
3. Eating raw can be as simplified as vegetable salads, fresh fruit, fruit or nut shakes and smoothies, nuts and seeds and a few sprouts. It can also be more gourmet by using a food processor to make sauces and dips, as well as a dehydrator to make crackers, cookies and veggie-nut patties.
4. Sweets can be enjoyed either as sweet, juicy fruit or in the form of sweet nut/seed candies and bars made from nut butters, carob, pure maple syrup, dates and/or coconut.

However you eat, as long as it's raw, you WILL LOSE WEIGHT!! Eat nutrient-dense foods, eliminate junk foods and "fattening" food from your diet, and you will lose weight. You will feel so good as you watch the pounds drop and your clothes begin to feel baggy. I have provided menus in Chapter X, my food diary for the first ten weeks so you can see the kinds of foods I ate for breakfast, lunch, dinner and snacks. During the first few weeks I feel I went overboard, due to enthusiasm, trying out new foods, making up new recipes. As the weeks went on, I simplified preparation time, the cost per meal and the number of ingredients used in a recipe, as well as the number of foods used per meal. This record will show you the variety of foods available and how to incorporate them into a daily eating plan.

It's very important, if you are very obese, under a doctor's care, taking medication or have any health problem or condition, to check with your doctor before beginning the "live foods" program. After six months on the "Live Foods Eating Plan" I have lost over 35 pounds, have gone from a size 12 to a size 6 or 8 and have increased my sense of well-being a hundred fold.

This is not a medically-based diet. It is an eating plan and is definitely more nutritious than the Standard American Diet (S.A.D.) that most of our country subsists on. It is a way of eating food in its natural form, unheated, to preserve most of the vitamins, minerals and enzymes naturally present in the whole, fresh food. It is based on the wise and accurate, long-time research of many raw foodists. I read and listen to them, then apply the recommendations to my own diet. We are each individuals and have individual tastes and preferences. By intuiting my own needs, I have experienced the healthful benefits, myself.

I began writing this book, foremost for myself, driven to stay motivated, to explore new ways of preparing food in appealing and tasty combinations. I felt like this was my last chance to try something different that might work. There is an old adage, "If you always do what you've always done, then you'll always get what you've always got". I didn't want to go through the rest of my life being overweight, prone to the same degenerative diseases that other Americans get, that are more attributable to diet and lifestyle (including lack of exercise, smoking, drinking alcohol, etc.) than to aging. I wanted to live life fully, feeling totally alive, energetic and healthy. I believe I'm on my way, and it just gets better and better.

As I excitedly created and tested recipes, after making the dish several times, tweaking the ingredients until I got it "right", I began thinking how much fun it would be to write a little recipe booklet and share it with friends and the community. I had a few Live Food Preparation classes and received a warm response. I felt I could save newcomers to Live Foods a lot of time, experimentation and energy if they were able to follow guidelines from the experiences of a relative newcomer, also. I could share my failures, recommendations and tried and true recipes.

I am not a fanatic about this. But, so far, I feel so good I may continue this path for a long time. Why go back to cooked food when I know now how healthy it is to eat this way? From medical doctors who make raw, living food their way of life because it is so life-supporting, to people with health concerns far greater than mine who are now glowing examples of what a simple change in eating habits can do to their physical, mental and emotional well-being, I have read too much to ever return to my old way of eating..

Three months into this way of eating, my husband and I were coming out of a movie, during which we ate or drank nothing. I had brought a grapefruit to peel and eat, but there were people sitting on each side of us and I felt it might out-smell the popcorn and maybe squirt someone sitting on either side, so I refrained from eating it. The point is, we were both starved, and it was well past dinnertime. After the movie I suggested we go across the street to the Thai restaurant and see if there was something we could take home. We went in and it smelled heavenly. We looked at the menu and there were only four salads on the menu. Everything else was cooked, deep-fried, stir-fried, steamed, grilled, broiled or baked. Looking at the description of the four salads I could see that there was only one that was raw--sliced cucumbers marinated in white vinegar and sugar. One salad used roasted peppers, one included bacon and cheese and a fatty-sounding dressing and the third one was a noodle salad with lots of soy sauce (probably MSG) and cold, steamed veggies.

Since I wasn't in the mood for cucumbers in vinegar and sugar, we headed for the nearest market where we loaded up on organic greens, raw nuts, some fruit and an uncooked olive dressing. I am sure that in the future, we will be able to go to a nice restaurant, ask the chef to prepare a fresh vegetable and greens salad and enjoy a vinegar and oil dressing on it or bring our own from home. At this point, I am enjoying my own concoctions much more than I feel I would at a restaurant. My ingredients are mostly organic, cut and diced in artistic ways, using only the foods I enjoy, which are a whole lot less expensive than what I would pay for some pale iceberg lettuce with a couple of tomato wedges.

Right now I am still on a roll, but aware that it is difficult to change one's eating habits. People will seek out a better way when they are ready. I am not playing the missionary game, set to convert everyone I meet. However, I get compliments and questions from all kinds of people about what am I doing to look so good, or how did I lose the weight. I try to answer these questions or refer them to a book or website where they will be able to locate the answer. I will talk about eating 'live' as long as a person is interested.

I do feel truly transformed. My body is shapely like it was when I was in my 30's. My skin is healthy-looking, my energy level is high and my joints aren't stiff and don't creak at all. I can hop out of bed in the morning without stretching. I am alert in the early morning as well as evening. I feel peaceful inside and go with the flow of whatever comes my way.

I predict all these things for you, too. Just give it a try for 5 weeks and then decide. Better yet, decide to go 100% raw for a day, then again for another day, and another. Notice how you feel. Listen to your body. Expect a little cleansing crisis in the beginning or withdrawal symptoms (headache, drowsiness, etc.) if you have been drinking caffeine in any form. But, day after day, you will begin to feel light and wonderful. This is my gift to you. Embrace it and embrace life. Life is too short to be living it halfway.

So, go for it. And, in the process, I will post my email address at the end of this book so that you can write me with any questions or difficulties you might encounter along the way. I would love to hear positive feedback too, about some new food you may have discovered or new recipe for a seed sauce you might have created, or an exciting cake or pie. The sky is the limit. The possibilities are infinite. Reach for the gold, uh, I mean apple!

Raw Energy

I'm a raw foodist, I do declare
And feelin' so high that I want to share
Why I don't eat eggs, dairy or meat.
In this poem, I'll tell you how I eat without heat.

On New Year's Day, I said, "I've had it! Enough!"
Trying to lose weight is way too tough.
I'd gained 40 pounds over the past 10 years
And couldn't lose an ounce, even cried some tears.

I'd been reading of people who ate everything raw
Uncooked, live food was their first law.
"Ever since the discovery of fire," they said,
Man's been scorching his food before he's fed.

He barbeques, boils, microwaves and bakes,
Steams and roasts everything from meat to cakes.
Even fruit is baked in a tart or pie.
Heating isn't healthy and I'll soon tell you why.

The animal kingdom eats raw and live
When in the wild, they usually thrive
A cow and an elephant are healthy eating grass
It's when a cow eats wheat that he fattens his
_ _ _.

For in fresh fruit and veggies, nuts and seeds
Are every nutrient a healthy body needs.
What you won't find in a burger and greasy french fries
In fruits, veggies and nuts, they're in abundant supplies.

But half of the vitamins are destroyed when food's fired.
Live enzymes are too, yet, for digestion are required.
But, when above 110°, raw food gets some heat,
Live enzymes are killed; it's not fit to eat.

Live enzymes are catalysts to build and repair
Damaged cells from the chemicals in junk food fare.
They help produce energy in every cell in our being
And increase our immune system in glands unseen.

But, best of all, live enzymes burn fat.
"Okay," I said, "I guess that's where it's at!"
These raw food people have really convinced me
But how and what do I eat? Pray, tell me I plea.

Well, for ten weeks I prepared raw food, made some messes.
Experimented freely, had failures and successes.
I steadily lost up to 25 pounds.
Yet, the food I ate was heaped up in mounds.

I didn't get hungry, nor did I feel deprived.
I turned back the clock, felt young and alive.
I slept less, worked hard and went to the gym
Soon my muscles were shapely and I looked fit and trim.

So if you want to lose weight and haven't been able
Just sit down with me at my 'live' foods table.
I'll serve you such hope you've never before seen.
Getting healthy and lean can be your most achievable dream.

Set a goal, love yourself, get ready to commit
It's work, but it's play, so decide you won't quit.
And as the weeks go by and you drop all that weight
Raw foods vs. cooked foods, you won't even debate.

by Lani A. Rossetta

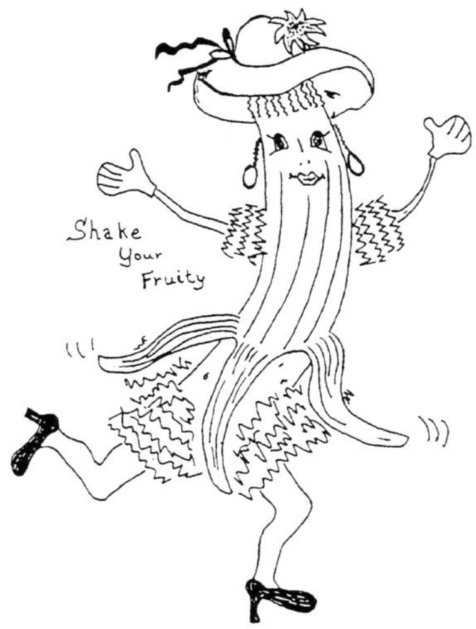

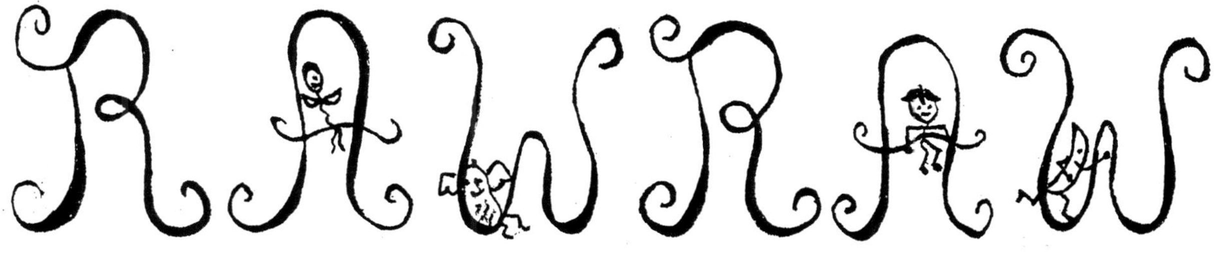

CHAPTER I
WHY LIVE FOODS?
(AND OTHER QUESTIONS)

1. Why Live Foods?

Live foods contain enzymes. As long as they haven't been heated above 118 degrees Fahrenheit, they are alive. Enzymes are catalysts for many processes that go on in every cell in your body. When a person eats a lot of processed foods, i.e., fast foods with salt, sugar and fat, the enzymes you were born with (metabolic and digestive) are recruited to help digest this food. Living food contains the enzymes necessary to process and assimilate the food they are contained in; i.e. amylase enzymes digest carbohydrates, lipases are enzymes that digest fats and proteases are enzymes that digest proteins. Since these enzymes are destroyed in the food by cooking, your own metabolic enzymes are used to digest the food.

Unless you eat a lot of fresh salads, raw veggies and fruits to provide these enzymes, you are depleting your own body's store of metabolic enzymes, thus contributing to low energy and aging processes. This usually happens from the age of 20 on. At age 50, because of a predominantly cooked food diet, your body's tissues contain greatly reduced enzymes, which are further decreased by being diverted to help digest the continued onslaught of cooked, lifeless food.

Some of the raw foods with a higher number of enzymes are: fresh dates, olives (sun-ripened), avocados, bananas, grapes, mangos, fresh raw figs, honey, germinated (soaked, then sprouted to only 1/4 inch long) seeds, grains and tree nuts. The soaking and sprouting process deactivates the enzyme inhibitors naturally present in the seed, grain or nut, thus increasing digestibility and assimilation.

Cooked foods have reduced vitamins, while live foods are like a vitamin in themselves, containing the vitamins we need in a balanced proportion, when consumed shortly after picking.

Raw foods are digested quickly and completely, with their own enzymes to help with the digestion and assimilation. This is like savings in the bank. You'll have plenty of energy and your immune system will be strong as you rid your body of toxins and poisons that were stored in your liver, fat cells, bloodstream, cells--toxins from drugs and stimulants like coffee, cigarettes, pesticides, etc. The list goes on and on. Think of all the processed food that adds sugar and salt for fillers, artificial food colorings and flavors, MSG and other possible allergens to your system. You will clear these out of your system and increase your health and well-being as well as your immune system. You will learn to prepare foods without sugar and salt, using herbs and sea vegetables. You will learn to appreciate the natural tastes of real foods rather than the salt or sugar that smothers the real flavors.

Live foods build a bridge between us and the earth, a connection between us and the sun and water that is required to grow these foods and a reminder of their gift to us of life-giving oxygen, a by-product of their own cycle which, in turn, uses our metabolic by-product, carbon dioxide. What a great symbiotic relationship.

Last, but not least, living foods contain the mysterious 'life force', called 'prana', 'Qi' and 'chi' in other cultures. The name I like is 'breath of life', a life force that presents itself in perfect form for humans and other living creatures on this earth to enjoy and nourish and sustain their own lives. Whatever you call it, may the 'life force' be with you!

2. What CAN I Eat?

You can eat anything you find in the produce aisle of your supermarket, farmer's market or food co-op. That means, any vegetable, fruit, nut, seed or grain that is on display in its natural, growing state. That means, you ignore the bottled or packaged salad dressings that are placed temptingly close to the washed, bags of salads. You also ignore any packaged croutons, dressing or dip mixes that might be hanging out by the carrots and celery. These are placed there for convenience, to remind you that you might want to dress up your veggies and fruits. But they AREN"T vegetables or fruits. You won't need to fret about eating foods that are processed, genetically engineered, hormone-filled, anti-biotic-filled, irradiated or full of pesticides when you buy Certified Organic whole foods. What a relief!

The nuts must be raw, not roasted, salted, smoked, etc. They can be shelled or in their shell. The seeds must be raw and able to sprout to prove they're still live. (More about this later). The beans must be whole and sproutable.

Dried fruits are okay as long as they aren't sulfured, sugared or candied. You will learn to dry your own.

The grains must be whole and can be hulled or unhulled, i.e. rolled oats have been separated from the germ and hulled and steamed, so are not raw; however, oat groats are usually raw. A live grain will sprout when soaked and most grains must be sprouted or at least soaked before incorporating into your diet.

You may make your own nut butters, or for convenience, buy raw, unpasteurized, nut and seed butters. That is all! But the above choices embrace 99% of everything growing in the fields, gardens and orchards for our consumption. Oh, yes, meat is out. You've probably been eating meat all your life. It won't hurt to leave it out for 10 weeks. And eggs are out. It's too dangerous to eat raw eggs, and for 10 weeks, you won't miss them. All dairy products are out, raw or not! Just for 10 weeks. Many vegetarians are vegans - they eat no eggs or dairy products and are as healthy as you or me. I've been 98% vegan for the past several years.

We can't forget the sea vegetables, which are full of ocean-bathed minerals, including calcium, plus some protein. There are many varieties to choose from and they are eaten in small quantities.

The only 'sugars' will be real, organic maple syrup, honey and dates. But have no fear, many sweet treats can be created from maple syrup or dates mixed with nuts, seeds and nut butters. And sweet fruits make a great dessert!

Of course there are herbs and low-salt or no-salt seasonings. We can't forget staples such as garlic, onions, lemons, fresh ginger and miso. Miso is a fermented soy or barley product and is not cooked or pasteurized. Tamari (a kind of soy sauce) is also fermented.

3. Can I Get Enough Vitamins and Minerals?

Consider this. If you are eating nothing but a variety of live fruits, vegetables, nuts, seeds, sprouted grains and beans, in other words, nutrient-dense foods, and eating until your appetite or stomach is satisfied, you can't help but get a variety of vitamins, minerals, carotenes, anti-oxidants and fiber. You will get protein (found in every real food), carbohydrates and healthy fats. Many cultures around the world eat this way. Sesame seeds, raw tahini (sesame seed butter), kale and collards rival milk for their calcium content and are assimilated better. Nuts and seeds contain magnesium, protein and good fats while fruits and vegetables are abundant in anti-oxidants and carotenes. B vitamins can be found in sprouted grains and nutritional yeast, and many trace minerals are present in the sea vegetables.

A live foods diet is high in fiber. Our teeth and digestive system were meant to chew and digest foods in their natural state. The more fruit, salads, nuts and seeds you can incorporate into your meals, the better. You will benefit from an abundance of vitamins, minerals and enzymes, which are greatly reduced in cooked meals. Not only your palate, but your plumbing will thank you!

Your body won't lack for anything, but if you wish, continue to take your daily multi-mineral-vitamin pill. Especially if you can't find an organic source for every purchase, you might wish to continue taking whatever supplements you were taking before, including a protein powder if you previously took one. More about this later, but you will be adding it to a Power Smoothie.

The only fats you will partake of besides avocados and flax seeds and the good fats found in olives, nuts and seeds, are olive oil and flax oil. You need the Omega 3's and 6's as well as the mono-unsaturated fats.

4. Can I Get Enough Protein?

Since every food contains some protein, you will most likely receive enough first-hand protein, especially if you vary your diet and eat something from each group every day (fruit, vegetables, nuts, seeds, sprouted grains, beans, seeds). (Second-hand protein is found in meat, i.e. the cow eats grass and grain so you are getting the protein second-hand if you eat meat.)

Sesame seeds are a complete protein and so is tahini, which is sesame seed butter. Soy beans are a complete protein. Wheat contains most essential amino acids, and when combined with a bean, makes a complete protein.

5. Can I Get Enough Calcium?

You will get to know the foods that contain a good amount of calcium. Some are sesame seeds, sea vegetables, kale and collards, almonds. Continue to take your own kind of calcium if you wish.

6. Do I Have to Be 100% Raw?

No, you do not, but if you are interested enough in this 10 week eating plan to buy this book and have tried every other diet under the sun with little success, you will find it very exciting and refreshing to eat fresh and live foods. You will delight in re-training or allowing your taste buds to savor the natural flavors in real foods. You will create magic out of mush. When you dehydrate a wet-looking patty for several hours and it comes out of the 'oven' looking and tasting as though it had been cooked, you will shake your head in amazement. Or when you pour a lumpy batter on a solid dehydrator sheet and watch it turn to crispy crackers, you'll wonder how it is possible. The same goes for bread-sprouted grains can transform into bread in a dehydrator.

So, if you are highly motivated to lose weight, to fit into your clothes better, to be healthier and more fit, then you will give it 100%, and that means going cold turkey. If you have under 10 pounds to lose, you might try eating 75-85% of your foods raw and live. You might eat raw for breakfast and lunch, then have steamed veggies with rice or potato along with a salad for the evening meal. There are many ways, but for the least temptation and guaranteed weight loss, go for it, 100%. The best part is you don't have to go up and down any of the other aisles. You don't have to make decisions about which cookie would be healthiest for you or which cracker to bring home with the least amount of saturated or hydrogenated fats. You'll be spared having to make many decisions. You'll feel freer when the only aisle you shop in is the produce aisle.

Just as in any new endeavor, take it one day at a time. Say to yourself, today I will eat only live, uncooked, whole foods. Or, for this meal, I will eat live foods, one day at a time. That is all we really have, anyway.

7. What About Exercise?

I bring you great news. When you exercise, your metabolism increases, you will burn fat rather than muscle and this continues many hours after you have stopped exercising. Yes, you have to exercise. You'll get rid of the toxins through healthy SWEAT, a very important route for eliminating toxins. Your skin will be healthier and rosier. Your heart, lungs and arteries will thank you. Your lymph system and circulatory system will be flowing in a way you haven't seen or felt for years. All it takes is at least 30 minutes a day. Take a walk, get on your treadmill, try a yoga class. Buy or rent some video tapes for yoga, step aerobics, lifting light weights. Join a gym and take an exercise class. Exercise when *convenient* in your day-morning, noon or night. Make it a healthy habit, something you do without questioning, like brushing your teeth.

Sometimes the energy of the class will be enough to keep you motivated. You will make new friends and enjoy seeing your exercise clothes get baggy as you lose inches as well as pounds. If you like to be alone or outside, invite a friend to take a walk with you. Walk your dog, push a stroller, or put a tape in your Walkman and listen through your headphones as you walk the mall, a bike path or around the block ten times. Park further from your destination so you can walk. Take stairs instead of the elevator. You know all of this.

The important thing is to have a support buddy to keep your motivation up. Even if they aren't eating the same foods, they can be available for exercise, for support and encouragement, and for cheering when they see your weight drop every week. Attitude is everything and you must stay motivated. The drop in the scales will keep you motivated.

8. Will Eating This Way Take All My Time?

Initially it might take a bit more time to prepare a big salad. You will soon learn shortcuts, like washing some of your produce before you put it away, or putting washed green onions, cucumber slices, radishes and cauliflower florets all in a covered, plastic container to slice or dice into a salad in no time. Carrots and red cabbage can be grated and put in a zip-lock baggie to use for several days. Your morning energy shake might take a bit more time than popping a bagel in the toaster and pouring a glass of juice. But when you realize the nutritional value of it and appreciate all the ingredients that go into it as well as the taste, it will be worth the extra 10 minutes it might take.

Also, it takes a bit more pre-planning. Remember when you were first living on your own and planned out your menus a few days in advance, before you shopped? You didn't? Well, I did and it was a lot of work at first. Eventually you learn to buy a variety of foods and to cook with what you have available. Sprouting beans or seeds for something you want to make will have to be planned a few days ahead of the recipe preparation, but they sprout themselves and grow. You just need to remember to water them daily.

And if you want a dehydrated patty or cookie, you can't just open a packaged mix and add liquids and put in the oven in 30 minutes. You have to plan ahead, because dehydrating takes many hours, but very little of your presence. You only need to check at certain intervals.

Yes, one will shop more often, because the food must be fresh and live, but it will soon become a habit, just as stopping for milk, bread and eggs was a 2 or 3 times a week routine. The longer I've been on this eating plan and grown accustomed to getting a variety of foods daily, the more I simplify and eat the whole fruit, nothing fancy, a great vegetable salad and maybe a smoothie or shake.

9. How Can I Feed My Family and Myself, Too?

Think simplicity! If you buy carrots to steam for your family, reserve some for yourself to eat raw! Steam corn on the cob for your family, while corn kernels sliced off the cob and placed in a salad for you will taste delicious! You'll learn to make your own uncooked salad dressings in an instant. Your family might enjoy them, too. If your family is going to enjoy baked potatoes with butter, you can quickly prepare Cauliflower Mash with flax oil and enjoy nearly the same taste. Everyone can have a green, vegetable salad, but make yours larger, the main course. Everyone can enjoy fruit for dessert and maybe a carob, maple, nut and seed bar. You'll adjust, they might enjoy some new sweet tastes, and everyone will be eating more nutritiously. Energy will be up, moods will be happy and calm. I truly believe we really *are* what we *eat.*

10. Do I Count Calories, Fat grams or Carbohydrates?

You won't want to. It takes up too much time because you will have such a variety of foods that you would be looking up the caloric, fat or carbohydrate value all day long. Use your common sense. If you are eating only fruits, vegetables, sprouted seeds, nuts and grains, it is highly unlikely that you will over-do the calories, fats or carbohydrates. Hypothetically, it's possible, but only if you eat 4 avocados, a cup of nuts, or 14 Fudgie Balls in one day, something you are unlikely to do. It might be beneficial for you, if you've forgotten all the wonderful vitamins and minerals present in whole foods, to get a food value book. If you are a man and interested in eating raw, you will be able to eat several avocados per day, 30-40 sun-ripened olives, if you wish, or several handfuls of soaked nuts.

David Wolfe, in his book, The Sun Food Diet Success System, has developed, over the course of years of observation and experience, a food triangle, similar to the food pyramids one sees in nutrition books, only this one does not have you count carbohydrate, protein or fat grams. Instead it focuses on three major areas of a live food eating plan: 1. green leafy vegetables (chlorophyll), 2. sweet, juicy fruits (sugars or carbohydrates), and 3. fatty foods, such as young coconut, olives, bananas, avocado. In the middle of the triangle are the rest of the fruits/vegetables. If one eats in equal percentages (by weight) from the three food descriptions in the corners of the triangle, then one will usually be balanced in their proteins, fats and carbohydrates. Obtain a copy of his book for more information on adjusting the triangle by different ratios, depending if you want to lose weight, gain weight, warm the body or cool it. This book contains a wealth of information on eating live, enzyme rich foods.

Articles in food magazines are often about the 30 best foods to protect against cancer, or the top 10 foods to prevent heart disease. These are fun because the same foods will be mentioned again and again for their protective value. You will see blueberries, bananas, avocados, broccoli, garlic, onions, oranges, cantaloupe and apples. Walnuts and almonds are often mentioned, also. There are recipes in this book using all of these highly nutritious foods, or they can be eaten just as they come off the plant-live and raw.

11. What About Coffee, Soda Pop and Wine?

Sorry, but you might surprise yourself by being able to go for 10 weeks without any of these caffeinated, carbonated or alcoholic drinks. You may get a withdrawal headache the first few days or be a bit lethargic in the morning, but that won't last for long. I thought I would miss my cafe' mochas, but I didn't miss them at all. I also saved quite a bit by not buying the mochas or eating out several times a week. I rewarded myself for sticking to this eating plan using the money I saved to buy myself something.

You can drink herbal tea as long as it isn't caffeinated. Steep the tea for 5 minutes, then drink when warm, not hot. You can drink warm miso soup. Heat water to under 105 degrees, then pour over a cup or small bowl containing a teaspoon of fermented miso paste. Add grated carrot, raw peas, thinly sliced green onion for additional flavor. (105 degrees is what your finger, dipped into the liquid can tolerate, a little warmer than a baby's bottle)

12. What About Fresh Air and Sunlight? Sunlight Daily for Vitamin D and Life Force

It is important to expose your skin to at least 20 minutes of sunlight daily to help your body produce vitamin D. Calcium requires vitamin D for good absorption. Enjoy the morning or late afternoon rays for maximum health and minimum damage from ultraviolet rays. Take glasses off if you wear them. Cup your hands and palm them over your eyes.

One Last Thing Your Emergency Bag

Keep an emergency stress-management bag with you at all times, or maybe make one up for your home, and one for on the road. Things to put in it would be whatever might deter your cravings for eating. Whatever would calm you and change your thinking. Examples are listed below.

1. your favorite cd's or tapes (i.e. meditation music, music to make you dance or move, an inspirational tape, audio tapes of workshops or lectures on inspirational subjects.
2. a reminder list of alternative things you can do besides eat (walk a treadmill, go to the gym, stretch over a ball, lift a few weights, do some squats, lunges or push-ups, jump on a mini-trampoline, write a letter to a friend, call a friend for support, go shopping at the mall and walk several laps while you're there)
3. inspirational books
4. video for belly dancing, yoga
5. a package of dried fruit or baggie of nuts or seeds
6. aromatherapy essential oils - peppermint, basil, and lemon are great to stop thinking about eating
7. a pair of walking shoes
8. a photo of you when you were at a good weight
9. a photo of you when you were overweight
10. a stretch band to do some stretches
11. bubble bath or good smelling bath salts/herbs to put in your bath

12. a project that you can work on with your hands, i.e. beading, knitting, crocheting, sewing, cross-stitch

13. a notebook for writing letters, beginning a book, jotting down an inspiration, writing a poem

14. your journal for writing your emotions and what event or stimulus caused the craving for eating something cooked, chocolate, sweet, full of caffeine, salt, fat, etc.

Are You Ready? Get Set! Go!

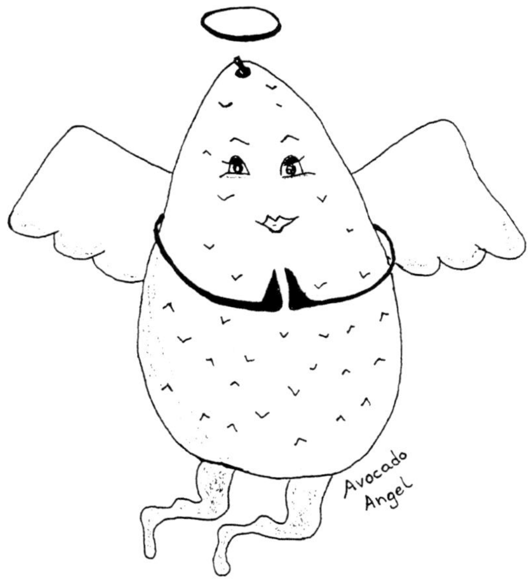

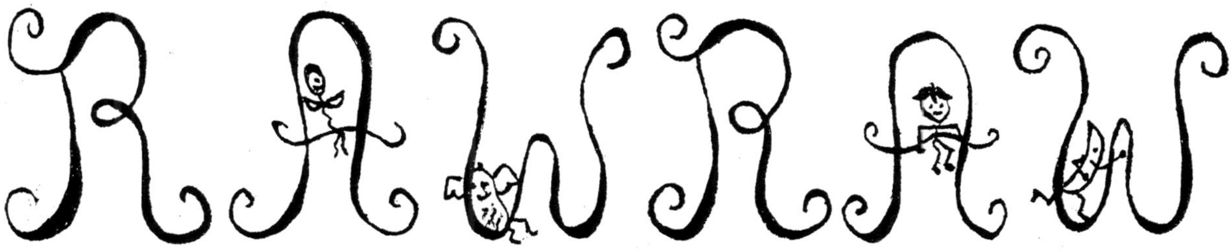

CHAPTER II
READY, GET SET, GO!

A. Basic Equipment

While eating "in the buff" for these 10 weeks, you will not be using the stovetop, oven or microwave. If all you had was a good, sharp knife, then you would probably be successful in eating raw, live foods. However, it might get a little boring. It's fun to play with textures, tastes, and the visual shapes of the fruits and vegetables. Following are some of the pieces of equipment that will make this journey a lot more interesting:

Several sharp knives, paring knife, serrated, perhaps a chef's rocker knife
A good vegetable peeler
An apple corer, slicer
A hand citrus juicer
A good cutting board, assigned only to your fruits, vegetables and nuts
A good grater

The following are nice to have but not necessary:

A fruit or vegetable spiral slicer - one that peels the fruit or veggie and/or slices it into spaghetti-like strands
A food chopper, one that will cut vegetables into "fries"
A garlic press, a ginger grater
A "Salad Shooter" or Mandoline - will slice or grate veggies in different thicknesses
An electric citrus juicer

Listed below are what I consider "essential" for your live food kitchen:

A blender
A food processor
A juicer
A dehydrator
A nut/seed grinder (coffee bean grinder)
A salad spinner (basically spins the excess water out of your rinsed greens and sprouts)

Miscellaneous equipment includes the following:

several sizes of colanders
several sizes of strainers
measuring cups, spoons
glass jars for soaking seeds, nuts and legumes (canning jars work nicely)
screens cut to fit the jars to be screwed on by the jar rings

B. Re-Filling Your Refrigerator

I happen to have two refrigerators, one in the kitchen and one in the family room. Truly, the grains, nuts and seeds last longer if they are refrigerated. I store these in labeled glass jars and plastic containers.

The carrots I buy in a 15 pound bag for juicing. The vegetable and fruit bins hold oranges, apples, dates, unsweetened coconut, greens and sprouts and all the salad ingredients. The more live foods you incorporate into your diet, the greater the need for a second refrigerator. If you have the room in your garage to put one in, it would be worth it. Used refrigerators can be found at a very low price.

Besides the great variety of fruits and vegetables, nuts and sunflower, flax and sesame seeds, be sure to always have on hand the following: lemons, miso (a fermented soybean, barley or wheat paste-both white and red), tamari sauce or Nama Shoyu, raw nut butters, raw tahini, raw carob powder, and unpasteurized apple cider vinegar.

Fruits: lemons, limes, oranges, grapefruit, apples, kiwi, mango, papaya, dates, coconut, jicama, tomatoes, etc.

Vegetables: avocados, sprouts, radishes, red cabbage, red leaf lettuce, mixed greens, red Swiss chard, kale, mini-carrots, cucumber, red bell pepper, jalapeño pepper, zucchini, yellow crookneck squash, butternut squash, yams or sweet potatoes, red onions, white onions, parsley, cilantro

Nuts: almonds, walnuts, pecans, pine nuts, Brazil nuts, filberts, cashews, macadamia

Seeds: sesame (hulled, but not bleached), sunflower (both hulled and unhulled), flax

Grains: millet, quinoa, barley, oat groats, hard wheatberries and soft wheatberries, amaranth, spelt, kamut, buckwheat (hulled and unhulled)

C. Preparing Your Pantry

Before getting started on your new eating plan, go through your cupboards and remove or isolate anything that is not raw or live. Make room in at least one cupboard to store some of your items. Since the food is live and raw, most of it will go into the refrigerator, but some things can be stored in the cupboard. Listed below are some of the items I frequently use:

raisins or any other dried, unsulphured fruit
nutritional yeast
soy-based protein powder (not a raw item, but one I felt I needed to continue. Mine has dried greens mixed in.)
seeds for sprouting: radish, alfalfa, clover (I usually buy these already sprouted), unhulled sunflower seeds for growing sunflower greens, unhulled buckwheat for growing buckwheat lettuce, hulled sunflower and buckwheat, hulled, brown sesame seeds
legumes: mung beans, adzuki, garbanzo beans (chickpeas), lentils
herbs: I buy either organic or non-irradiated by the bulk: Herbamare (sea salt and herbs), Veg-It (herb blend), All Purpose Seasoning - Frontier brand (dehyd. onion, parsley, lemon peel, basil, thyme, dehyd. garlic, celery, red bell pepper, citric acid, freeze-dried whole lemon)
other herbs: basil, thyme, oregano, cayenne pepper, paprika, onion granules, garlic granules, dried garlic bulbs, chili powder, sage, rosemary
Poultry Seasoning - Frontier brand (sage, thyme, dehyd. onion, marjoram, black pepper, celery seed, red pepper)
5 Spice Powder - (fennel, cinnamon, cloves, star anise, white pepper)
allspice, cardamom, nutmeg, cinnamon
vanilla and almond extracts
Celtic salt
Nori sheets (seaweed dried in sheets for making Super Sushi or in small snack size pieces for crumbling over salads or eating as a snack), purchase untoasted
Kelp or Dulse powder or flakes - for sprinkling on patties or salads for added minerals
Hijiki - a sea vegetable - very good in miso soup or on salads when soaked and rinsed
Wakame - same as above

Edible Flowers to Garnish Loaves, Patties, Salads

Add a real sensory, artistic and gourmet touch to your meals by using edible flowers in your salads, or garnishing loaves, patties, etc. with colorful, tasty, unique flowers. All your senses will be activated and enhanced: sight, smell, taste, touch. The colors are beautiful and the idea of eating flowers is not something you see in your everyday restaurant. Try it and enjoy the subtle aromas and tastes. Remember never to eat flowers that have been treated with pesticides.

This is a partial list of some flowers that are edible:

basil blossoms - mild basil flavor; use in soups, salads
borage petals - cucumber flavor; use in beverages, soups, salads - remove the base if using the flower whole
calendula petals - slight tart taste. Use petals, discard the center. Use in soups, salads
chamomile
chives - lavender blossoms taste of chives; use in soups, salads, spreads
chrysanthemum
cilantro - white blossoms taste like the leaf, only milder; use in spreads, salads
citrus blossoms
cornflower petals
courgette blossoms (zucchini)
daylily - use in soups, salads
dianthus petals
dill flowers
elderflowers
English daisy flowers - light, floral taste, use petals in salads or soups
fuschia petals
geranium,
gladiola
hibiscus petals
honeysuckle
Johnny jump-up - petals taste slightly green, herbaceous; use in salads
lavender blossoms
lemon - strong citrus flavor; use to flavor drinks, freeze into ice cubes for lemonade
lily petals
marigold petals
mustard - strong, peppery taste; use in salads, soups or spreads

nasturtium petals - peppery with watercress flavor; use in salads or to flavor cider vinegar
orange and apple blossoms
pansies
rocket flowers
rose petals - salads
squash blossoms
strawberry blossoms
sunflower petals
tulip petals
viola heads
violet heads
wild rose petals
yucca flowers

Don't forget wild greens. They are rich in vitamins and minerals, full of chlorophyll and can be delicious. In the Pacific Northwest, where I live, one can easily hike a trail and locate miner's lettuce, purslane, malva and lamb's quarters. Almost everyone has dandelions in their grass, and the young, spring leaves are very good additions to your salad.

My friend and I walked my backyard labyrinth during the Spring Equinox. We were observing the herbs I have planted around the inner ring of the labyrinth. Martha noticed that 3 of the plants had miner's lettuce growing around them. She remarked to me about it and I was literally delighted. On coming out of the labyrinth, I looked at some plants outside the labyrinth on the east side. There, along a wall, the compost bin and by the walnut tree, were miner's lettuce plants, thick as any clover or grass. It's a beautiful plant with cup-shaped or heart-shaped leaves, and flowers that grow out of the center of the leaves. The stems are long and succulent. All parts of the lettuce are edible, sweet, juicy and delicious. I have been cutting some daily and adding to my Power Smoothie and salads.

Visit your library or nearest agricultural station and find out the local, edible plants in your area. You may be as lucky as I was to find some growing in your own back yard.

Tip: Perform the art of live food preparation and serving the way you would expect an artist to paint--with enthusiasm and love for the people who will enjoy the completed dish. If you are stressed, it will be reflected in the vibrations of the meal you prepare. Be calm, gentle and loving, so as to bring food to the table with peaceful and harmonious vibrations.

D. One Way to Approach These 10 Weeks

Always check with your doctor first before going on any weight-reducing program. Show him/her the menus, eating plan and recommended foods.

Decide to go cold turkey into raw foods. You are on an adventure, probably doing something totally different and foreign to any diet or eating plan you've ever attempted before. Yet, at the same time, you are already familiar with eating raw, uncooked fruits, green salads, juices and fruit shakes, nuts and seeds. So, rather than fretting about what you must do without for 10 weeks, focus on the variety of foods you *CAN* eat. You're going to do fine. You will succeed. And the weight will drop off like butter melting off the corn cob. Tell yourself you are now ready to release the weight forever.

This is the path I chose because I couldn't merely cut down on my regular eating plan. To cut from 4 mochas a week to 1 or 2 wouldn't work for me. Or to cut down on breads and starches wouldn't work, because I was already eating very little breads. I had a sweet tooth and desired to cut out sweets entirely. I have been a vegetarian for 27 years, rarely eating dairy foods and fish, maybe 2-3 times a year in the past few years. So it wasn't much of a leap for me to try totally uncooked, living foods.

It's too difficult when you are at so many social occasions to say "no" when you are offered organic chocolate brownies or home-baked bread. I always had to have a piece, then another, and you know how that goes. There will always be a social occasion. There will always be tempting treats to try. So, I decided if I really wanted to lose weight and become healthier, I would try the raw foods route for 10 weeks. If you choose this path, you will lose weight consistently for 10 weeks. Remember, you can't overdo it on raw foods unless you eat 10 mangoes at one sitting or snack on raw nuts and seeds all day long. I don't recommend either. If you follow my menus exactly, or substitute similar things, you WILL lose weight. I was 155 pounds when I began eating live foods (had crept up to 160 in the weeks prior to getting back to 155 pounds). I lost a total of <u>25</u> pounds (averaging 2 pounds a week after the initial 5 pound loss the first week), and I am still losing at the time of this writing (about 1 pound a week). My weight will stabilize by itself. I am confident of that. If not, I'll increase the food intake to maintain my weight. However, I have not been hungry since beginning this eating plan, other than a healthy appetite to eat!

Remember the old adage, *"If you always do what you've always done, then you'll always get what you've always got."* Make this your mantra and repeat it daily, especially when motivation is low. Remember what didn't work in the past and why. Memorize this and make up a little tune so you can sing it when you walk, when you exercise and when in the grocery store. This Live Foods Eating Plan is different from any 'diet' you've ever been on, yet strangely familiar. You already have eaten practically every food on this list, just maybe not raw, nor in the combinations found in some of the recipes. You may not have eaten every meal raw, but now you will. So, you see, the food is not unfamiliar, just the manner in which it is put together for a 10 week eating plan.

A Step-by-Step Plan for Families Going Raw

Note: Before undertaking a 100% raw eating program with the younger children in your family, please purchase a good book on how to raise healthy, vegan (no flesh foods, no dairy, no eggs) children. There are certain nutritional needs that young, growing children must meet for good development (calcium, protein, etc.) and only a good book from a knowledgeable and experienced author will give you the real scoop. Do your research!

1. Begin very gradually, especially if the children are used to their junk food snacks, cold cereals, instant soups, cookies, crackers, and candy. One way to begin is to decide to replace all afternoon snacks with fruit, veggie or nut snacks. (See # 5, #6 and #7 below.) (See Chapter V Snacks, for other ideas for snacks for on-the-go!)

2. Another way is to replace just one meal with only raw foods-the easiest of these being breakfast: Have fresh fruit available in a fruit bowl on the dining table for the children to choose what they like. Teach them how to make a fruit shake or smoothie. At night they can cut up the bananas or wash the strawberries and freeze them in covered containers. In the morning they can use the citrus juicer to juice oranges, add some sunflower seeds, a little nutritional yeast, frozen bananas, strawberries or any other berry to the blender and blend for a filling, delicious, nutritious meal.

3. Show them how to make a glass of nut milk for their smoothie-simply by blending 1/4 cup of almonds in a cup of water, straining, then pouring back into the blender to make a fruit shake. They can learn to appreciate 'milk' that doesn't come from a cow. And sweet 'yogurt' that doesn't come from a cow.

4. Begin by replacing the sweetened, fruit juices with the whole fruit. Help the children get used to peeling an orange, slicing an apple or eating it whole, or using an electric citrus juicer for oranges and grapefruits.

5. Keep a covered, plastic container in the refrigerator filled at all times with any of the following: sliced, fresh pineapple, orange boats, grapes, kiwi slices, apples, halved and cored. This provides something instantly for the children when they are hungry after school and don't think they have time to peel an orange themselves. They'll be more likely to eat fruit or veggies, if they are already washed and ready for them. Have a container of raw nut butter for them to dip them in or a fruit sauce.

6. Keep a separate, covered, plastic container with fresh, washed veggies. The kids can go to the container, take out what they want and add a dip or dressing that is freshly made for an instant snack. Container might include: olives, celery slices, radishes, mini-carrots, cucumber circles, jicama slices or cubes, sweet red pepper strips, green onions.

7. Have a few refrigerated jars or containers of raw nuts: almonds, sunflower seeds, cashews, pecans, walnuts. The children can mix these with raisins, sunflower seed sprouts or dried apples and bananas in zip lock bags, which will be instantly available when they are hungry for crunch.

8. Have fruit leather available for snacks. The children, with the help of a dehydrator, might enjoy making their favorite fruit leathers, or dried cherries, mango slices, pineapple, grapes.

9. Freeze green, purple grapes, cherries on toothpicks for "jawbreakers", a sweet substitute for popsicles. Popsicles can be made from any fresh juice.

10. Never nag the children to eat raw. First they must acquire a taste for anything you offer. Don't be afraid to try exotic fresh fruits. Some are very creamy and tasty, i.e. cherimoya, and the children might be willing to try something different. When their friends come over and eat some of the snacks and think they are cool, your children might be more willing to continue to eat for better health.

11. Give your children some recipes for some sweet nut balls. Using raw tahini or almond butter, some honey or maple syrup, a few chopped nuts or raisins, and a little carob powder, your children might become very creative in inventing their own nut ball concoctions. When refrigerated or frozen, they make tasty snacks to eat at home or take with them to school or sports practice.

12. When it comes to eating salads, sometimes children are very picky about certain vegetables or salad ingredients. Though it takes more bowls (buy the small, plastic, covered containers), you might try a variety of several salad ingredients, and let the children pick and choose what they want to put on top of their lettuce. (Have 2-3 different kinds of lettuces, too.) This way, they can feel they are in charge and free to choose a few ingredients. Compare it to a salad bar at a buffet. Make up a couple of salad dressings that they like.

13. Sometimes cucumbers and zucchini, tomatoes and other salad ingredients aren't especially appealing when cut in slices and circles. Try grating the zucchini, yellow squash and other ingredients that will make it much easier to chew and eat in their salad. Sometimes, they won't even recognize the ingredient (i.e. radish grated with carrots and zucchini). Again, sometimes when the veggies are cut into matchsticks they are more fun to eat as finger foods with a dip.

14. When you purchase your fresh ingredients, take time to wash the greens, the vegetables, before refrigerating. When clean and available, your children will be more likely to make up a salad or use the veggies with a dip. Using your food processor with grater attachment, grate some carrots, zucchini and beets, (each separately), then place in zip-lock bags, so they will be readily available to use when dinner comes around and everyone is hungry. (Purchase a salad spinner: a must-have, to rinse off the water from your washed greens and sprouts. Children will enjoy turning the crank to 'spin' off the extra water. This prolongs the life of the greens and keeps them from getting 'rust' on them.)

15. Allow children to shop with you and get used to shopping only the produce aisle, along with the bins of nuts, seeds and dried fruit. Try packages of different dried fruits if you don't have a food dehydrator. (Food dehydrators are available at your discount department stores for less than $40 dollars.

16. Take time to discuss with your children how they might be feeling about this; how they might be noticing they have more energy, less cravings for sweets, feeling better, sleeping better, awakening more easily in the morning. Accept whatever they might express and discuss as a family.

17. Teach each child how to prepare their favorite sauce or dressing. All they usually need is a blender. They will feel like they are contributing to the health and appetite of the family.

18. Since some of the preparation takes a bit of time and one's kitchen can get messy in a hurry, teach your children to rinse the utensils, bowls, etc. and place in dish washer as part of their clean-up routine. It saves time and energy for cleaning up after a meal.

19. Teach the older children how to use the food processor for grating, chopping and mixing. Show them how to use a knife properly and safely. Make sure you have one cutting board reserved only for fruits and vegetables and always keep it rinsed and clean.

20. Make planning meals (shakes, smoothies, salads, sauces, main dishes) a family affair. Provide the ingredients for their favorite foods and make them often. Write down their ideas for menus and meals. It will make shopping a pleasant experience.

21. Initially, keep the raw meal or snacks something that is done at home. When kids are out with their friends, don't enforce the raw foods. It is a goal (yours) that soon, with the candy, cookies, and crackers out of the house, that they will come to appreciate the sweet tastes of fresh fruit, the enjoyable tastes of eating their own nut and seed balls, and making up their own shakes.

22. Try to encourage raw food eating and make it fun. Read passages from books that the children can understand and assimilate into the reasoning that the family is trying to eat fresher, livelier whole foods. Talk about the body and what it needs for good nutrition. Make the teaching, discussion short. There will be plenty of opportunities to bring this subject up without over-doing it. Think of the 'battle' you have with the advertisements, billboards and commercials of over-salted, over-sugared, over-fat, processed foods. It's like trying to fight city hall. You can only do your best by being a good example for your children and educating them about the value of living foods.

23. Form a support group of other families who want their children to eat better (even if not entirely raw). Have meetings, dinner parties, snack parties, any get-together where there is a sharing of food. Be sure to have some board games or fun times for the children so they learn to associate good times with their food.

24. Finally, try to keep it simple, both in the beginning and throughout. Make it a voluntary thing, but something you believe in wholeheartedly. Make small changes, one step at a time, even if it's just to

introduce one new fruit a week, or one new vegetable a week. Try not to get overwhelmed by going too fast, too soon. It will just defeat the purpose and might alienate your children from your new way of eating.

An Exercise-Food Log is Essential

Keep an exercise-food log. Buy an inexpensive notebook and begin to keep track of the following things, daily:

a. date and day of week
b. next to that, record your weight, weighing when you first arise after voiding, with no clothes on.
c. next to your weight, write in the exercise you did for the day, even if it's a 15 minute walk or parking 10 minutes away from your work and walking to work; climbing the stairs instead of taking the elevator, etc.
d. below the line containing the above information write B. on one line for breakfast, S. for snack, L. for lunch, S. for snack, D. for dinner and S. for snack. Leave a couple of lines for each meal or snack.
e. write in everything you ate, even if 2 almonds, or a T. of raisins. Write it in.
f. at the bottom of the page, write any comments you might make:

1. how you feel physically
2. how you feel mentally
3. how you feel emotionally
4. what your craving was, or trigger for a craving? (if you had a craving that day)
5. if you had a craving, did you try anything in your Emergency Bag first?

g. write comments next to your meal if it was filling, nourishing, tasty, something to try again, and so forth. Especially if it was satisfying until you needed or wanted a snack or the next meal.

Looking back weekly in your diary or journal will be very helpful to pinpoint the time of day or stress that set off a particular craving for comfort food - i.e. chocolate, junk food, fast food, and so on. You will begin to develop more useful strategies to ward off that craving, until one day it will disappear altogether, or at least will not bring you to the point of going off your eating plan. Even if you do, remember that all is not lost. If you eat a cooked food once or twice in a week, don't beat up on yourself. Be gentle and know that you are improving your health, losing weight and gaining energy each and every day.

Please be aware of some of the difficulties you might encounter during the first ten weeks:

1. Cravings for your comfort foods - sweet, salty, sour, crunchy, smooth, creamy
2. Peer pressure - invitations to lunch, dinner out, parties, food at the office, etc.
3. Previous addictions, or, more accurately, old habits
4. Detoxification symptoms - feeling less than your best as your body releases toxins
5. Emotional highs and lows due to daily stresses
6. Motivation, commitment, desire or lack of - enlist a support buddy for you to talk to

Tip: Nutritional yeast provides the B vitamin complex, 16 amino acids and 18 important minerals. My preference is in the form of flakes rather than powder. Store in a tightly-covered container and use frequently in shakes, drinks, loaves, seed sauces and patties.

Dry Brushing of Skin

During this 10 week eating period of live foods with live enzymes, consider dry brushing your skin daily. It will help remove toxins that are trying to get out, is great for the circulation and will give your skin a radiant glow. Choose a brush that feels good to your skin, long-handled preferred. Brush from the toes upwards toward the heart. You can try long strokes (i.e. from top of foot to knee) or short circular strokes as you move upward. You can go around your lower leg, front to back, before moving upwards, or brush the entire front of your body, then brush the back side. When you are brushing your neck, shoulders and arms go toward the heart. Soon, you will notice your skin is smooth and youthful-looking. Brushing also helps move cellulite, slough off old dead skin and stimulate circulation and lymph flow.

It is better to brush in the morning when you are getting your energy up for a full day's work. However, sometimes I dry brush in the shower before I turn on the shower, then wash the dead skin and toxins away.

Foods Good to Apply to the Skin

Eyes - Apply cucumber slices directly over closed eyes for refreshing tired eyes; also, try herbal tea bags.

Body Scrub - Apply sea salt with a damp washcloth and give your entire body a rub down. Shower off.

For the face -

1. quick face 'lift' - When you're through juicing a lemon, rub the inside of the lemon, pulp and all onto your face. Leave on 10-15 minutes before rinsing. Gently bleaches dark spots.
2. quick moisturizer - When you've sliced the avocado out of its half-shell, rub the inside of the half shell onto your face, using that last bit of avocado. Great for the skin.
3. facial scrub - Grind 1/4 cup almonds in blender. Add enough fresh pineapple, papaya or melon to make a creamy consistency.
4. face mask - Blend 1/2 banana with 1 T. lemon juice and 1 t. sesame oil. Leave on for 15 minutes, then rinse away.
5. face mask - Mash 1/2 avocado with 1 t. lemon juice and 1 t. honey for a lovely green face mask.
6. face refresher - Blend 1/4 cup cucumbers with a little avocado for a refreshing mask.
7. face toner - Mash 2-3 ripe strawberries and apply to face. Rinse after 15 minutes.

Total Body Moisturizer - Use sesame oil for any part of your body that needs oil--your hair, elbows, soles of feet, between the toes, your face, arms.

Daily Mantra or Affirmation

My daily mantra, one I repeat several times a day is:

Live Foods! Plant Foods!
Raw! Raw! Raw!

Okay, go ahead and repeat it 3 or 4 times. Doesn't that sound like a cheer that will keep you motivated? Will it keep you interested in learning all you can about nature's laws, the first one being to eat foods raw? Eat raw and natural, close to the earth, food from the sun. Try this one:

Foods that are raw, will leave you in awe!
Foods that are alive, will make you thrive!

Here's another one I like:

Every day, in every way,
I am feeling healthy and fit!
or - I am releasing my fat!
or - I am letting go of my old body!
or - I am becoming my most perfect weight!

Now, go create your own!!

Let Me Introduce You . . .

The guides, angels and spirits you will see on the next page are your own personal helpers to assist you during the next ten weeks. You will find them throughout this book -- coaching you, supporting you, reminding you to keep the faith. They will encourage you to blend those Power Smoothies, enjoy the greens in your salad, and have a little fun while doing it. Ta Da!

Introducing Avocado Angel, Fruit Fairy, Greens Goddess, Let's Salsa, Shake Your Fruity and last, but not least, the Sprout Spirits. Please talk to them and listen to them. They are here to keep you motivated. If you see or feel the presence of any other guides or spirits, use any empty space to draw in your own. Now, let's get going with the recipes!

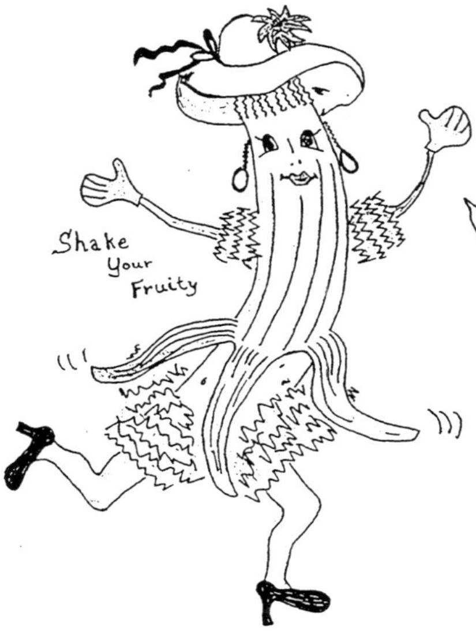

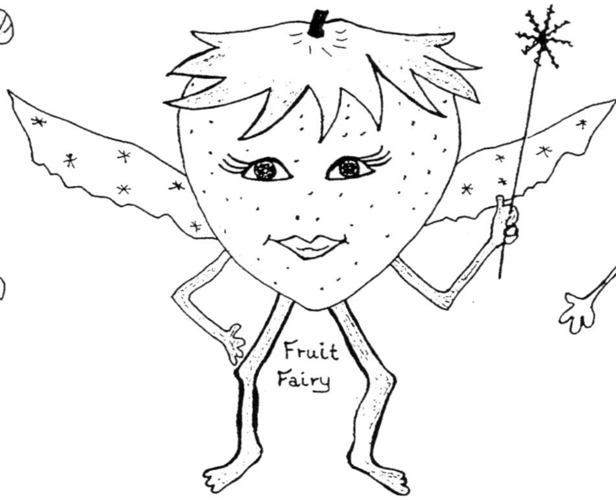

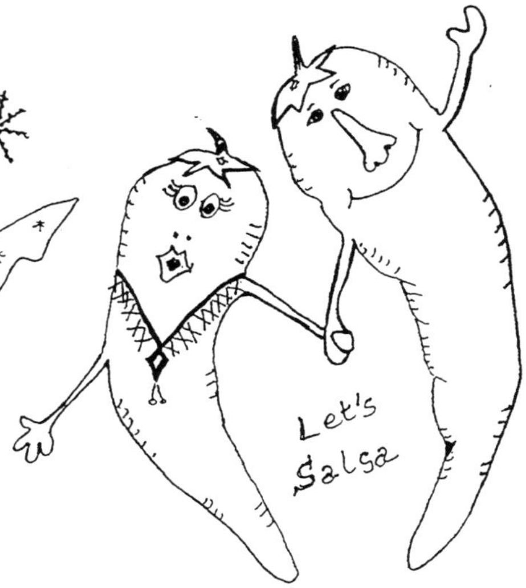

RAWSOME RECIPES

RAW! RAW! RAW!

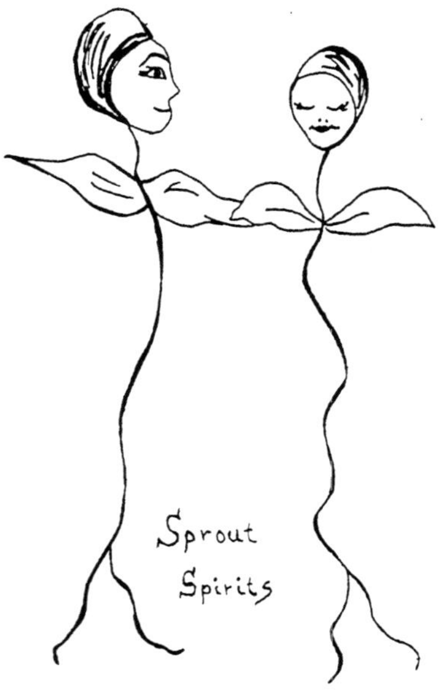

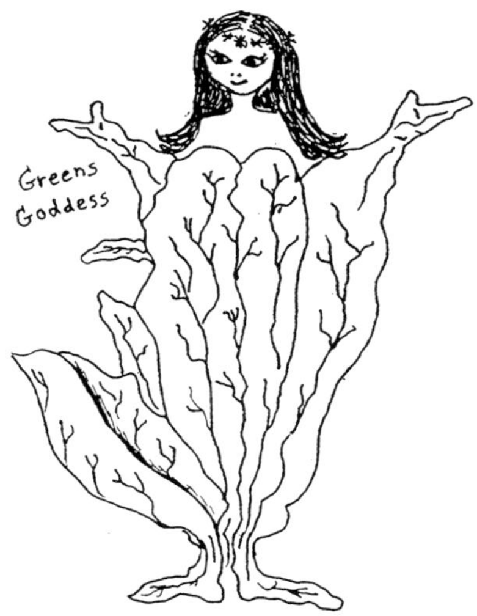

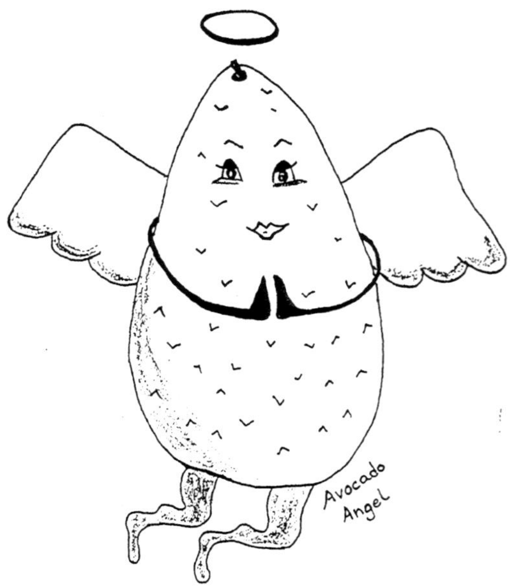

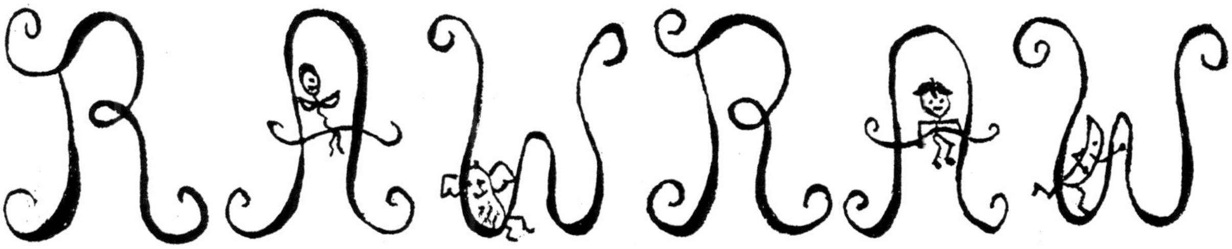

CHAPTER III
DRINK TO YOUR HEALTH
(JUICES, SMOOTHIES, SHAKES, MILKS)

Juices

Juices play an important role when one is eating raw foods. Freshly juiced, raw, organic vegetables, sprouts and fruit contain live enzymes, anti-oxidants, beta carotene, vitamins and minerals in concentrated form. It is easier sometimes to juice your greens than to chop them and eat them--greens such as kale, collards, cabbage and green pepper. There is nothing tastier than a glass of fresh, pineapple juice. It doesn't begin to compare with canned pineapple juice. An 8 oz. glass of carrot juice can be made from 3 to 4 carrots. Add greens to the carrot juice for a great drink. The nutrients are dense and calories minimal if you mostly stick to vegetable juices. It's better than taking a vitamin pill. Today, juicers can be found in many discount department stores for under $100. Give juices a chance. It's possible to make some of these in a Vita-Mix blender, but you are drinking the pulp; therefore, digestion takes longer, whereas the pure juice is excellent on your digestive system when fasting.

Liquid Sunshine

2 oranges
4 small carrots
4 T. raw sunflower seeds or sunflower seed sprouts

Juice the two oranges in a citrus juicer. Pour into blender. Juice the carrots in a juicer. Add juice to blender. Add sunflower seeds and blend. Drink slowly.

Variation: Juice 4-6 carrots. Pour into tall glass and sip very slowly, almost chewing the juice.

Rainbow Blend

4 carrots
1 stalk celery
1 beet

Scrub veggies well. Put them through your juicer. Stir, sip, and enjoy.

Apple-Ginger Zinger

4 apples - choose your favorite
1/2 lemon, juiced
1/4" slice of peeled ginger root

Juice the lemon and pour into a blender. Juice the apples along with the ginger. Blend in a blender until smooth.

Salute to the Sun

Juice 1 lemon. Add water to fill a tall glass and stir in 1 t. maple syrup.

Green Spiral

1 c. water
1 c. fresh carrot, orange or pineapple juice
1 t. Spirulina
1 T. lemon juice

Blend and serve chilled.

Tip: Watermelon – great juice for kidneys . High in potassium and is alkalizing. Balances pH.

Liver Detoxifying Drink

16 oz. pure, distilled water
1/2 lemon, juiced
1-2 T. organic maple syrup
1/8 t. cayenne pepper

In a tall glass pour 16 oz. pure, warm water, the juice of 1/2 lemon, 1-2 T. real maple syrup and 1/8 t. cayenne pepper. Stir and drink. Repeat this drink 4-5 times, evenly spaced throughout the day. Do this on a day when you eat nothing else, or when you drink nothing but green vegetable juices, i.e. a combination of celery, cucumber, spinach and green pepper.

Jubilation Celebration

2 cups carrot juice
5 almonds, soaked overnight
2 T. sunflower seed sprouts
1 T. sesame seeds, ground
4 apple juice cubes (frozen in ice cube trays)

Blend all ingredients in blender except apple juice cubes. Slowly add the cubes and blend well. Toast with this cocktail when going off a fast, before eating solid food again.

Aloha Nui

In blend, blend the following fresh juices:
1/2 cup pineapple juice
1/4 cup carrot juice
1/4 cup orange juice
juice from 1/2 papaya

Divide into glasses and squeeze a little lime juice into each glass. Place a slice of lime on the rim of each glass.

Vitamin Energizer

1 handful wheat grass

Cut a small handful of wheat grass into 2 inch pieces. Place in a blender with a little water and blend. Strain and pour the green juice into a pitcher of fresh pineapple juice. Stir well. This is a lovely, mint-green juice that contains a balanced ratio of vitamins and minerals.

V-6 Wake Up

2 tomatoes, chopped
2-3 T. olive oil
1 t. powdered kelp or dulse
1 garlic clove (optional)
1/4 t. onion granules
dash cayenne

Blend all together in a blender. Add a sprig of parsley and drink. Good liver cleanser

Pineapple Plus Energy Drinks

Each drink makes approximately four servings. Juice 1 whole, peeled pineapple. Place in a blender. Add any of the ingredient combinations below. Blend with the pineapple juice, then enjoy as is or strain and pour into glasses. (Optional: any of the ingredients listed below can be juiced with the pineapple, thus eliminating the necessity for straining, if you don't want a thick drink)

1. Pineapple juice + 7-10 fresh spinach leaves and 1 handful rinsed, alfalfa sprouts
2. Pineapple juice + 1/2 to 1 avocado, 2 T. coconut, 1 banana
3. Pineapple juice + 1 papaya, 2 bananas, 1 avocado, 1/2 lime, juiced
4. Pineapple juice + 1-2 oz. wheat grass juice.
5. Pineapple juice + 8 oz. apple juice, 1 banana, 6-8 oz. carrot juice, 1 T. ground sunflower seed sprouts

Herbal Teas

I like to buy a variety of herbal teas, all decaffeinated. I enjoy Good Earth's Sweet & Spicy tea, Yogi Tea's Detox tea and Celestial Seasonings Ginger-Ease Wellness tea.

Healthy Soda Pop

Mix 3-4 oz. of your favorite fresh fruit juice with 8-10 oz. of sparkling mineral water for a bubbly drink.

Rejuvelac

1. Wash 1 cup of soft wheatberries.
2. Soak in a quart jar for 24 hours in 2 cups of pure water.
3. Pour off water into a glass container and stand at room temperature for 1 day.
4. This is rejuvelac. It should taste lemony. Refrigerate.

Use in place of the water in seed yogurts, cheeses, sauces and dressings. Use the soaked wheatberries for growing wheat grass OR add more water to the berries and soak 24 hours for a second batch of rejuvelac.

Tip: Put some wheat grass in distilled water to add back life force and minerals to the water for drinking. You are adding liquid sunshine.

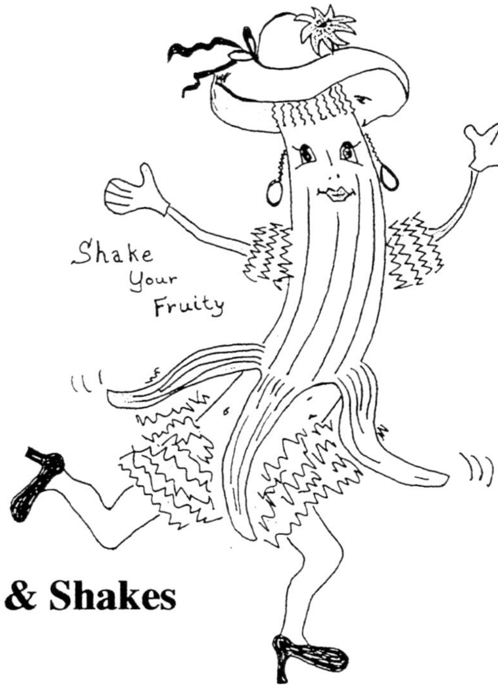

Smoothies & Shakes

Super Smoothies

For most fruit smoothies use frozen banana chunks as a sweetener and thickener. Simply peel ripe bananas, cut into thirds and freeze in a covered container. Usually the equivalent of one banana will thicken a 14 oz. smoothie or shake.

Variation: any fresh fruit may be frozen in chunks, whole (as in berries) or pureed and then frozen in ice cube trays for thickening and flavoring a shake or smoothie.

Try fresh or frozen berries, grapes, cantaloupe, pears, peaches, cherries, fresh avocados or pineapple, papaya, nectarines, strawberries, blueberries. Fresh fruit may be added along with any frozen fruit or bananas. Add any fresh fruit juice for a delicious smoothie.

1. Pour juice in blender (about 12-14 oz. for 2 servings)
2. Add frozen fruit to juice
3. Blend until smooth and thick
4. Try adding a pinch or dash of one of the following spices: cinnamon, nutmeg, mace, anise, cardamom, mint, grated lemon or orange peel.

Tip: Make lemon ice cubes. Mix 2 cups of water with 1/2 cup lemon juice. Pour into ice cube trays. Add a sliver of lemon peel to each cube. Keeps juice cold while adding zing! Can also be used to cool warm teas.

Carob-Date

Blend 4 pitted dates, 1/2 t. vanilla, 1 T. tahini, 1 T. unsweetened coconut, 2 t. raw carob powder, 8-10 oz. apple juice and enough frozen banana chunks to make desired thickness.

Pineapple Berry

Blend pineapple juice with frozen strawberries.

Beta Blue Smoothie

In blender place:

juice from 2 oranges
1 frozen banana
1/2 to 1 cup frozen mixed berries

Blend until smooth and thick.

Variation: In place of orange juice, use 10-12 ounces almond, sesame or sunflower seed milk.

Mellow Yellow

Blend 3 parts apple juice, 3 parts orange juice, 1 part pineapple juice, a few squeezes of fresh lemon juice and enough frozen banana chunks to make thick.

Tip: In a glass of water, place a paper-thin slice of lemon. It looks elegant and makes the water taste sweet and delicious.

Strawberry Smoothie

Blend all together until smooth and thick:

1/3 cup cashews
1 3/4 cups water
1 t. flax seed, ground
6-10 frozen strawberries
1/4 cup frozen blueberries
1/4 t. cinnamon

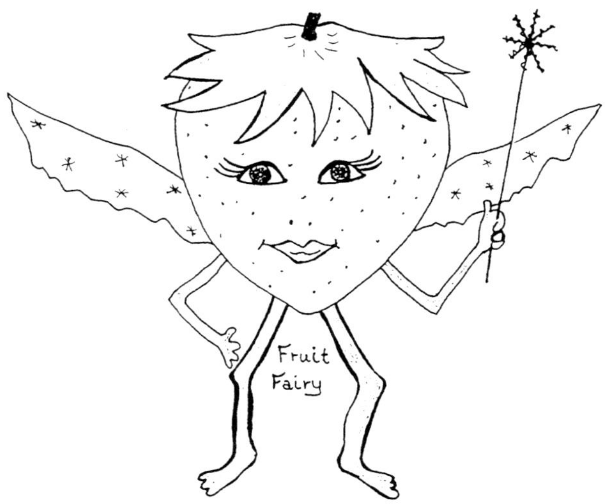

Power Smoothie - Power Shake

Place the following in a blender:

Juice from 2 oranges plus 1/4 cup water (vitamin C, antioxidants)

1 scoop of your favorite protein powder (my protein powder has soy isoflavones, spirulina, barley grass, chlorophyll and kelp)

1/2 frozen, peeled banana (potassium)

2-3 organic kale leaves (calcium, carotenes)

1/4 cup frozen blueberries (antioxidants, folic acid)

Blend until smooth. This smoothie, which has lovely orange, green and blue layers of color will be green or purple when blended. Pour into a tall glass and slowly sip, trying to chew any pieces of orange, banana or kale in the smoothie.

Additions: 1 T. nutritional yeast (protein and B vitamins)

1 T. lecithin granules

1-2 T. sunflower seeds or sunflower seed sprouts

1 T. flax seeds, ground first in nut/seed grinder (Omega 3 and 6 essential fatty acids, fiber)

Variation: In place of kale add 1-2 Romaine lettuce leaves, 1 large red Swiss chard leaf, a handful of washed alfalfa or clover sprouts, miner's lettuce, a collard leaf.

Variation: Substitute fresh or frozen strawberries, black berries or mixed berries for the blueberries.

Variation: Substitute a nut or seed milk for the orange juice. Omit the green leaves, add 1 t. spirulina and call it your Power Shake.

This should keep you satisfied until lunch. Great for high-stress days, or before or after working out! Although this Power Shake or Smoothie is filling and complete, it is usually drunk in the morning as a great way to begin the day, but sometimes it is my main meal.

Peach Smoothie

In a blender, place 1 peach, sliced, 1 cup of orange juice, enough frozen banana chunks to make a thick smoothie.

Tip: When there is an abundance of ripe fruit in your fruit bowl, puree and freeze in ice cube trays, to be used later in fruit shakes or smoothies. OR puree and pour onto solid dehydrator sheets and dehydrate until chewy. Roll up and wrap in plastic wrap for a tasty fruit leather snack.

Sunny Apple Flax Seed Smoothie

Blend the following until smooth and thick:

1/2 cup sunflower seed sprouts
1 cup fresh apple juice
2 frozen bananas
1 T. flax seed, ground
1 T. almonds, ground
1 t. cinnamon
1 t. cardamom

La Luna Freeze

In a blender, blend:

4 oz. green tea - (2 green tea bags steeped for 5 minutes in hot water, then cooled)
4 oz. pineapple juice
4 oz. orange juice
enough ice cubes to blend into an icy freeze. (Can add a little powdered Stevia for sweetness)

Variation: May add a few frozen banana chunks along with the ice cubes for sweetness

Tip: Watch for specials on any kind of fresh, ripe fruit and buy in quantity. Wash, peel, core and freeze on a cookie sheet, then store in covered container in freezer.

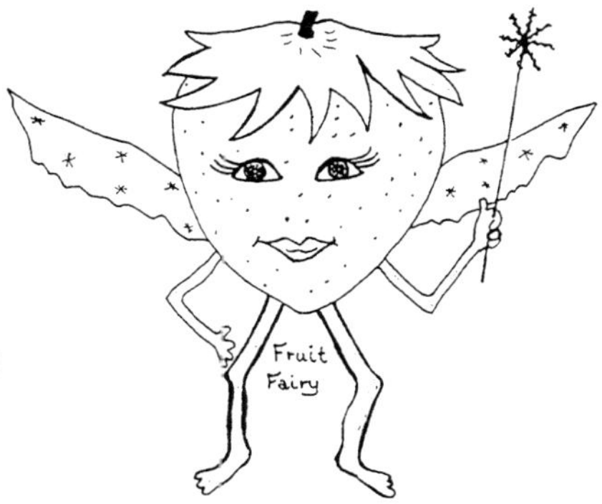

Super Milk Shakes

1. For 2 servings, fill blender with 14-16 oz. of any nut or seed milk.
2. Add frozen banana chunks for desired thickness.
3. Add any of the following sweeteners and flavorings: 1-2 T. of real maple syrup, carob powder, tahini or any nut or seed butter, 1/2 to 1 t. of pure vanilla or almond extract, Almond-Cinnamon Mixture.
4. For high energy shakes add any of the following: 1-2 T. of figs, dates, raisins, cranberries, sunflower seed sprouts, unsweetened coconut, ground flax seed, walnuts, almonds, cashews, ground sesame seeds, nutritional yeast
5. Blend all until thick and smooth.

Got a Date with a Fig Shake

Blend the ingredients below in a blender:

3-4 fresh figs, chopped
1 cup nut milk
4-5 Medjool dates or twice as many smaller dates
1 t. vanilla
2-3 chunks frozen bananas
3-4 ice cubes

Carob-Banana Shake

Fill blender container with 16 oz. nut or seed milk. Add frozen banana chunks, 1 t. vanilla extract, 1 T. carob powder and 1 T. real maple syrup. Blend until smooth.

Thick and Fruity

Fill blender container with 16 oz. milk. Add frozen banana chunks and any frozen or fresh fruit. Blend until thick and smooth.

Janet's Bone Builder Shake

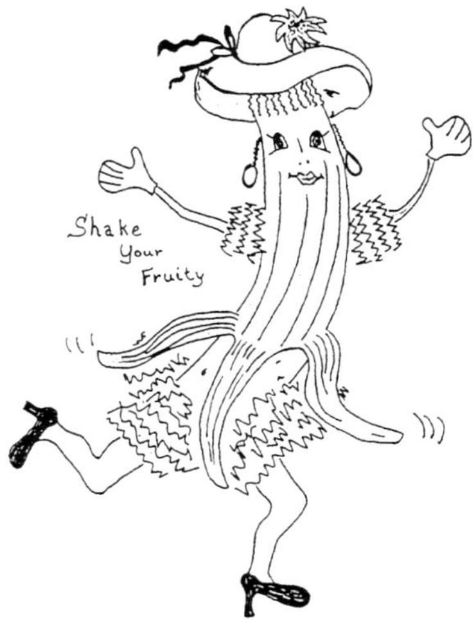

In a blender, blend the following ingredients well:

1 cup milk - almond, cashew, soy (transition food)

1 banana, peeled

1/2 cup fresh fruit - cherries, cantaloupe, etc.

1 T. flax seed oil

1 t. calcium citrate powder

2 T. yogurt - seed, nut or soy

Variation: May add 1 T. carob powder for a chocolate flavor

Earthshaking Shake

Blend the following until smooth and thick:

12 oz. almond milk

1 frozen banana

1 - 2 t. Almond Cinnamon mixture

Variation: For a chocolate shake, omit the Almond Cinnamon mixture and add 2 T. carob powder.

Variation: Try sesame seed milk in place of almond milk.

Variation: Substitute frozen strawberries for the banana and omit the almond-cinnamon mix.

Variation: Add 2-3 Medjool dates to the shake.

Almond-Cinnamon Mixture

To 1 cup of finely ground, raw almonds, stir in 1 T. cinnamon. Store in a covered glass jar in the refrigerator. This mixture not only tastes good in shakes but can be sprinkled on fruit, yogurts, or as a topping on a fruit pie.

Nut and Seed Milks

Generic Nut Milk

Generic recipe for nut and seed milks: To 1 cup of raw nuts (blanched, if desired), slowly add 3-4 cups of water while blending at high speed. Blend until smooth; then add 1 T. maple syrup and a pinch of salt. Blend again, strain (for smoothness-optional), and refrigerate in a covered jar. May be used in any of the shakes or in yogurts. When using seeds, use 1/2 cup seeds with 1/2 cup nuts. Almond-Cashew or Almond-Sesame are good combinations. Yield: 4 cups milk

Almond Milk for One or Two People

1/4 cup almonds
2 cups water

Soak almonds overnight. Remove skins. Blend with water. Strain and refrigerate.
Optional: For sweetness, add 1 t. pure maple syrup.

A Quart of Almond Milk

3/4 cup raw almonds, soaked in water 18 hours (save soak water for smoothies)
1/4 cup raisins, soaked just until softened
5 cups distilled water

Rinse soaked almonds and place in blender. Do the same with the raisins. Pour in 1 cup of distilled water and blend until smooth. Add another cup of water and blend for at least one minute. Strain into a pitcher. Pour in the remainder of the water, then strain again. Refrigerate, covered until ready to use. Reserve almond meal for part of your breakfast muesli.

Variation: In place of raisins, add 1 T. pure maple syrup with the final cups of water.

Sesame Seed Milk

To make sesame seed milk: Use the unbleached, brown, hulled sesame seeds.

In a blender blend the following:

1/2 cup sesame seeds, (hulled but not bleached), soaked
4 cups water

Blend well, then strain. Refrigerate.

Sweet Cashew-Date Milk

1 cup cashews
2 1/2 cups water
4 T. chopped dates
1/2 t. cinnamon

Blend cashews and water in a blender. Add dates and cinnamon and blend again. Pour into a covered jar and chill. Tastes great to drink or pour on sprouted grain cereal, such as Captain Buckwheat Crunch.

Variation: Substitute 1/2 cup orange or apple juice for 1/2 cup water.

Tip: Using organic flax seeds in your shakes or smoothies adds important fatty acids: omega 3's and omega 6's, essential to your daily diet. Whenever using flax seeds, remember to grind just before using, as they can quickly turn rancid if ground ahead of time. Ground flax seed is a great laxative, also. Just 2 T. of flax seeds, ground in a seed mill and added to your shakes will thicken the shake and take care of your needs for fiber and a bowel movement.

Warm Carob Cocoa

Warm 2 cups of any nut or seed milk. Do not exceed 105 degrees. Mix 3 T. carob powder, 3 T. maple syrup, 1 T. olive or flax oil and 1/2 t. vanilla extract. Add to warm milk.

Warm Carob "Mocha-Chai"

2 tea bags (Good Earth Original - Sweet & Spicy Herb Tea)
16 oz. water, brought to a boil, then removed from heat.

Steep two tea bags in 16 oz. hot water for under 5 minutes. Cool slightly.
8 oz. almond milk (Using a scant 1/4 cup soaked almonds, blend 8 oz. water in blender, then strain.
To 8 oz. almond milk add:
1 rounded t. raw carob powder
1 t. pure maple syrup

Remove tea bags from water. Pour tea in large, 24 oz. mug or thermal mug. Pour in sweetened milk. Stir and enjoy. Mocha-Chai will be warm, but not hot.

Variation: Wait until mixture cools, then pour over a tall glass of ice cubes for a refreshing, cool drink.

(Good Earth Sweet & Spicy Herb Tea contains: Rooibos (Masai), Rose Hips, Chamomile, Cinnamon, Lemongrass, Peppermint, Papaya Leaf, Anise, Orange Peel, Ginger)

This is a delicious drink and quick to make for a day when you want something warm.

Tip: To blanch almonds, bring water to boil. Take off burner and wait a minute. Pour hot water over almonds for about 10-15 seconds. Then pinch the almond at pointed end and the skin will usually pop off. If not, scratch it a little and it will easily peel off.

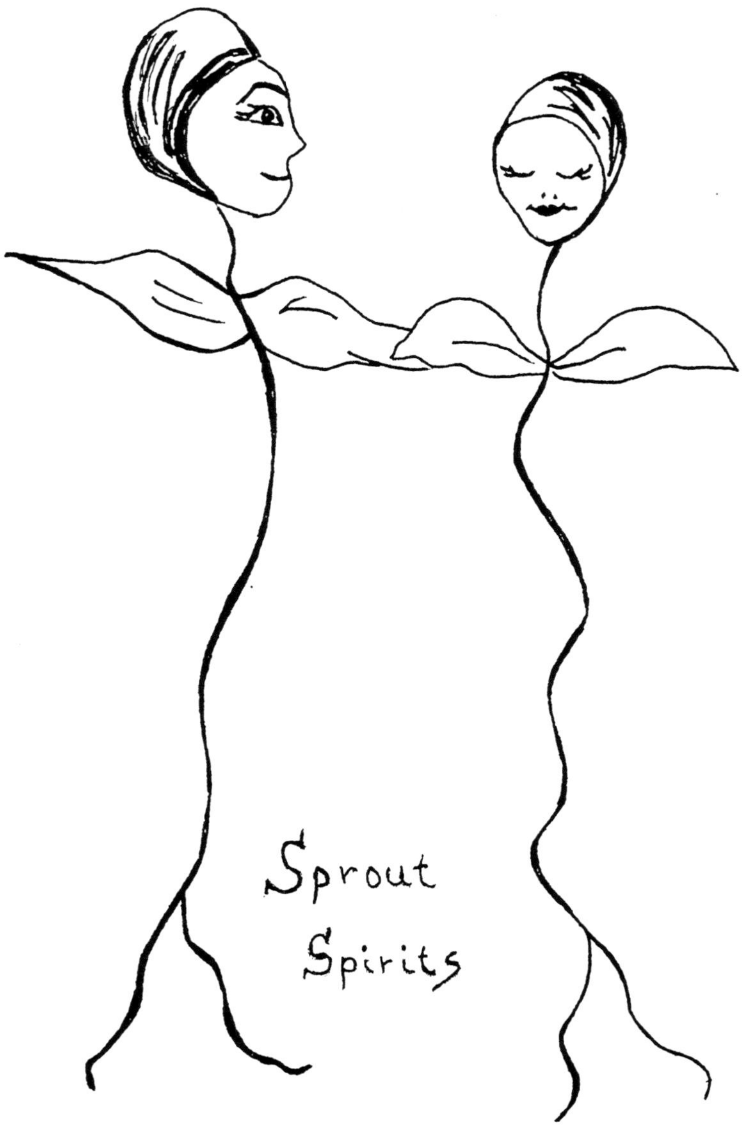
Sprout
Spirits

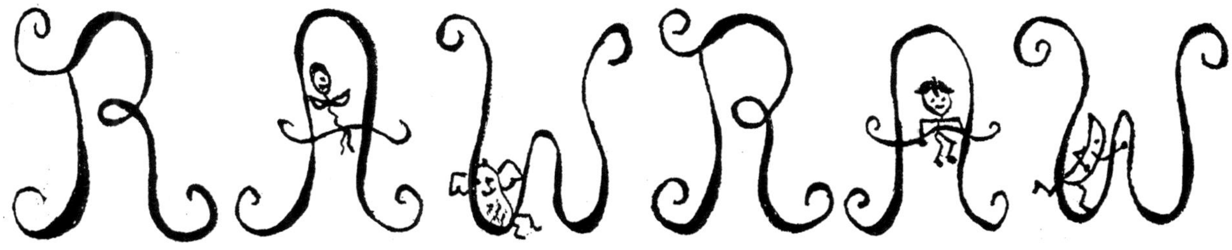

CHAPTER IV
LIVELY SPROUTS!

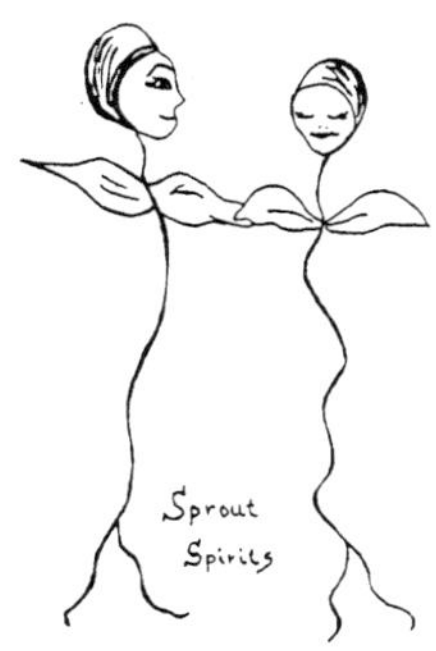

Seeds, Nuts, Beans, Grains

Wanted: A live vegetable that grows in any climate, rivals meat in nutritional value and tomatoes in vitamin C, matures in 4-7 days, does not require soil, has no waste, is pesticide-free, can be eaten raw and stays crisp in salads.

Found: Sprouts - sprouted from nuts, seeds, grains and beans. Sprouts are live foods, have a high degree of enzyme activity, are easy to digest, rich in vitamins, minerals and protein. All of the life-giving properties of the seed are released into the sprout and multiplied many times to provide minerals, vitamins and protein. They are a real powerhouse of nutrition. All you need is a jar, some seeds, water and a light source.

Why Sprout?

If someone told you that you could eat an organic salad every day of the year for only pennies per pound of greens, that the greens were grown without soil, and could be grown on your own kitchen counter or window sill, you might think they were out of their mind! But sprouts are those greens and they live up to every bit of hype you might ever have read about them. They can be grown indoors, any season of the year, any location in the country as long as you keep the temperature of the room you are growing them in the same moderate temperature that you like to live in - between 68 and 75 degrees. They will grow in a warmer temperature but may sometimes spoil if not rinsed often or if over-heated. They grow from seed to your salad bowl in less than a week.

Nutritionally, sprouts are amazing. Once the seed, bean, or grains are sprouted, they increase multi-fold in vitamins, protein and other important substances than if they had remained a bean or grain for cooking. Sunflower seed sprouts have much more nutrition than raw sunflower seeds, as do wheat sprouts contain more vitamins than the grain. Look at some of these statistics:

Alfalfa sprouts have more chlorophyll than cabbage, kale, parsley or spinach.
Alfalfa, clover, radish and sunflower sprouts are about 4% protein. Iceberg lettuce has only .8%.
Soybean and lentil sprouts each contain over 25% protein, while meat has 19% and eggs, 13%.

Needless to say, the fat in grain sprouts is highly digestible and won't go rancid. The anti-oxidants, vitamins, phytochemicals, minerals and live enzymes are what make sprouts a valuable addition to your salads.

Think about this: Sprouts are readily available, no pesticides are involved, no genetic engineering, no irradiation, are economical, low in calories and fat, high in energy and are environmentally conservative, i.e. require little water to grow, no soil and no special equipment. Doesn't that sound like a dream salad ingredient? You don't have to get in your car and shop at the grocery store. They are a kitchen counter vegetable.

Love them, talk to them, water them, rinse them and watch them grow.

What to Sprout

The following seeds, nuts, beans, grains are what I sprouted during these 10 weeks.

alfalfa sprouts
red clover sprouts
radish sprouts
mung, lentil and adzuki bean sprouts - sprouted together for salad toppings and Curried Lentil-Mung-Adzuki Sprout Salad
garbanzo beans (chickpeas) - for Oregon Hummus
lentils - for Sprouted Lentil Patties
wheatberries (both hard red and soft white) - for cereal, patties and dehydrated bread
oat groats
barley, hulled
kamut - for bread

spelt - for bread
quinoa - for Tabouleh, salad topping, cereal with fruit
buckwheat groats - for Captain Buckwheat Crunch, Crisp Buckwheat Frisbees, nut and seed balls
buckwheat (unhulled) for growing buckwheat lettuce
sunflower seeds (hulled) - for anything and everything
sunflower seeds (unhulled) - for growing sunflower greens

My Favorites

Favorite sprouting/soaking seeds are: alfalfa, clover, sunflower seed, radish, flax
Favorite beans are: chickpeas, soy, lentil - both brown and red, mung, adzuki
Favorite grains are: wheat, quinoa, buckwheat
Favorite nuts to soak and/or sprout are: almond, pecans, walnuts, pine nuts, cashews, macadamias
Favorite greens or lettuces to sprout and grow are: wheat grass, sunflower lettuce (from unhulled sunflower seeds), and buckwheat lettuce (from unhulled buckwheat)

Equipment for Sprouting

Do you have some glass jars? Wide mouth canning jars are ideal, because you can cut a circle of plastic screening to fit the top of the jar and hold it in place with the jar ring screwed over it. It is essential to have a jar with some kind of permeable cover. Old pantyhose, cut a few inches bigger than the jar top and attached with a rubber band to the jar, also works well. Cheesecloth will work but is slightly more difficult to rinse and clean than window screen or nylon. A third alternative is not to have a lid at all, but to rinse the seeds in the jar, then pour in a strainer or colander to drain; later, when sprouting, they can sit in the colander or strainer and be rinsed under the faucet.

So, you will need: glass jars, nylon or screening and a rubber band or jar ring, strainers, colander, a dish towel to cover (when they soak or need to be in the dark), a sunny windowsill or counter top for greening the sprouts that want to green, and good quality sprouting seeds, for human consumption. Get these at a farmer's market or food co-op.

With one exception, which I will describe when I get to them, certain greens, such as wheat grass, buckwheat lettuce and sunflower greens, do better when grown in soil. The taste of the buckwheat lettuce and sunflower greens is worth the effort, resulting in something beautiful, tasty and nutritious to add to your salad or other raw food dishes. The wheat grass juice is also worth the effort for the added enzymes and nutritional value. Wheat grass requires a meat grinder or wheat grass juicer to juice, which is the best way to consume the wheat grass.

How to Sprout

I like to think of sprouts as lively and friendly. They do their best to please you as you grow them from the seed to the sprout. I've even experimented between two jars of alfalfa sprouts, both just beginning to sprout, both grown from the same batch of seeds. I wanted to see if my intention for one jar of sprouts to grow faster than the other would cause that to happen. So for several days, I watered each of them equally, rinsed the same and put in the sunlight only 2 feet from each other. The one jar was left alone except for this care. The other jar, I placed my hands above and focused on these little sprouts growing fast and tall. I sent them love and intention to grow tall and healthy. Sure enough, much to my surprise, the jar that received the most attention reached maturity before the other jar. Well, I guess I wasn't that surprised, because it's been proven to be true with laboratory rats. Many of us know that plants respond to love and attention. Even a person who thinks he doesn't have a green thumb can be successful growing sprouts. Besides being easy to grow, every seed, bean or grain grows a different sprout and it is fun to watch them change, both inside and out. Kind of like we do, grow and develop from within and without.

All beans, grains, sprout seeds, and nuts (sometimes) are soaked before using in raw food preparation. The reason to soak the nuts is for easier assimilation and digestion. The beans, since they won't be cooked, will be soaked, then sprouted. Grains will become more digestible, also, when sprouted.

A general rule of thumb for how long to grow the sprouts is to sprout until the little, white sprout tail is about as long as the seed it grows from, and no longer. For example, sunflower seed sprouts will tend to taste bitter if the sprout grows longer than the seed. Garbanzo beans (chickpeas) will be ready for use after growing about 1/4" inch of a tail; the same for adzuki beans and lentils. Almonds will begin to grow a nub of a tail in a couple of days after soaking, and that is enough. Most beans, nuts and grains are grown in the dark. Mung beans are also grown in the dark with a weighted plate placed in the jar. The exception to this rule of thumb are mung bean sprouts and the alfalfa-radish-clover-broccoli seed type sprouts. These will green up (or remain white if mung sprouts) and grow many, many times longer than the seed they grow out of.

Tip: Soybeans are a complete protein. They are low in carbohydrates, rich in calcium, phosphorous and iron and contain vitamins A, B, C, D, E, and K. They are also rich in lecithin--nature's cholesterol emulsifier. Include them sprouted in salads, sandwich spreads, patties or loaves. They are harder to digest than other beans, but use them sparingly for the food value they contain. Always sprout them until the sprout is almost the length of the bean. Grind in a food processor, using the 'S' blade.

Steps to Growing Beautiful, Lively Sprouts

1. Rinse the seeds, beans, grains (not nuts, except cashews).

2. Place in a jar and cover with water.

3. Cover with a towel or place in a dark corner for several hours. I usually begin the soak before I go to bed and rinse off the water in the morning to begin the sprouting process..

4. Once the water is rinsed, the jar is turned upside down at about a 45 degree angle to further drain and be rinsed 2-3 times a day. Continue this until the sprouts begin to grow. Then follow directions for each individual sprout as to whether to green it, or refrigerate it once the tail is the length of the seed.

5. Alfalfa-radish-clover-broccoli seed sprouts are all sprouted in the sun (after the soak) for several more days until they look like the ones you purchase in the store.

To Fluff Up Sprouts Before Eating

To prepare for use, take a small handful of sprouts and place in a bowl of cold water. Separate the sprouts by swishing your hand in the water. Soon, all the little brown hulls will come to the surface and usually cling to the sides of the bowl. Gently scoop the sprouts out of the water, avoiding the hulls and place in your salad spinner or in a colander to drain and dry before placing in your salads.

That's it! Nothing more. At the end of this Chapter is a sprouting chart to show soak times, days for sprouting, length of sprout, etc.

Sunflower Seed Sprouts

Wash raw, hulled sunflower seeds in a colander. Pick out the dark ones. Place seeds in a glass jar and fill with water. Soak overnight. In morning, drain and rinse. Drain again and cover colander with a paper towel or cloth. Rinse twice more during the day, draining well after each rinse. By evening a tiny sprout will be forming. You may refrigerate at this point or continue to rinse and drain three times a day for one more day until sprout is as long as seed, but no longer. Refrigerate. Use in drinks, salads, puddings, yogurt, soups and on Buckwheat Frisbees. They taste crunchy, nutty and are high in protein and other nutrients.

Tip: Add a handful of radish or cabbage sprouts to a green salad for an extra zing. Be sure to sprout with seeds meant for sprouting. Seeds for planting are often chemically treated with fungicides.

Wheat Sprouts

Soak wheatberries overnight. In the morning, drain, rinse and drain again. Repeat two or three times a day for two days or until sprout is just the length of the grain. Refrigerate until ready to use. Chewy and surprisingly sweet. Use in salads, sprout candies, cookies.

Mixed Sprouts

1. Soak 1/4 cup of a mixture of adzuki, lentil and mung beans overnight.
2. In the morning, drain, rinse, drain and invert. Rinse twice daily. By the second or third day, when the sprouts are as long as the beans, rinse, drain and refrigerate.

Variation: Substitute soy beans for mung beans.

Sprout Combos

1. In a quart jar, soak 2 T. of alfalfa and/or red clover seeds OR 4 T. of wheatberries, OR 4 T. lentil-mung-adzuki beans, in at least 1 cup of water.
2. Soak overnight, drain, invert and rinse 2-3 times per day until the sprout is as long as the bean, grain or seed. Exception: alfalfa or clover sprouts should be placed in the sun to green when the sprout begins to grow.

Mung Sprouts

For salads, mung beans can be sprouted in 2-3 days to a sweet, tender crunchiness. But for a mung sprout pasta and other dishes you may want them nice and plump. If you just let them grow longer, the roots would get long and spindly instead of plump.

Try following these directions for crisp bean sprouts

1. Soak 1/3 cup of mung beans in a large 1 1/2 quart jar overnight.
2. In the morning rinse, drain and keep the jar inverted all day, with a piece of nylon screen or cheesecloth attached to the opening with a rubber band. Rinse 3 times the first day.
3. On the second day, rinse, drain, and place a tall, thin jar filled with water inside the jar or bowl of sprouts (this serves as a weight). Rinse only mornings and evenings now, and keep sprouts in a dark corner of your kitchen or cover with a dish towel. Make sure to drain well after each rinse.
4. By the fifth or sixth day, your bean sprouts will be long, thick, white, crispy and delicious.
5. Store any extras in a paper or plastic bag or container in the refrigerator.

Wheat grass

Sprout wheatberries in same manner as sunflower seeds. Then place in a shallow tray which has one to two inches of very damp plant soil mixture. Cover with damp paper towels; uncover to rinse once daily. When stalk grows, remove towels, expose to light and water daily until grass is dark green and about seven inches tall. Cut at base for juicing.

This spring, in our garden area, we discovered a patch of wheat grass. I had thrown out some old wheatberries that I hadn't even attempted to sprout. Well, you guessed it! A large patch of wheat grass is growing in our garden. I cut a bunch, then cut some young dandelion leaves and juiced them in my greens machine. It's a delicious and powerful drink, rich in chlorophyll and vitamins and minerals. However, one shouldn't drink more than a few ounces at a time. Drink on an empty stomach and be prepared for a zing! It's a very detoxifying drink and must be drunk in small amounts.

One day, after drinking some wheat grass juice, I was getting ready to go to exercise class. It's a good thing I decided to brush my teeth, because when I looked in the mirror, I saw a very green wheat grass juice moustache attached to my upper lip, curving upwards at the edges. Wouldn't that be great to be driving along and noticing a big billboard with a picture of a healthy, fit person, with a green moustache, holding a glass of wheat grass juice and saying, "Got wheat grass juice?" It certainly is a lot healthier than a billboard with some athlete promoting milk and saying, "Got milk?"

Buckwheat or Sunflower Lettuce

To grow pesticide-free buckwheat or sunflower lettuce indoors, year-round: Soak 2 cups unhulled buckwheat or 2 cups unhulled sunflower seeds overnight in a large jar with 3 cups water. In the morning, rinse, then spread on a tray of soil. Cover for 2-3 days. When sprouts are up, uncover and place in sunny window. When leaves grow and plants are 4-6 inches in height, harvest by cutting at the base of the stems. Rinse so that hulls will drop off before eating. Use in salads. Sweet and delicious.

Tip: Twelve pounds of powdered wheat grass contain more vitamins than 340 pounds of veggies and fruits --more veggies and fruits than the average person can eat in a year. So dry those leftover sprouts and whea tgrass, and powder them in a blender. Store in a cool cupboard in a covered container.

Mini-Lesson on Soaking Most Nuts and Seeds Before Eating

1. Soak all grains and beans before eating, preferably sprout them, according to each individual grain or bean. This releases the inhibitors and makes them more digestible.

2. Most nuts and seeds are soaked overnight in a glass jar in plenty of water.

3. If desiring to sprout, then rinse in the morning, put a piece of screen or cheesecloth over the top with a rubber band and tip upside down on a rack.

4. Rinse 3x a day until the sprout is as long as the seed, bean, grain or nut it comes from. Exception would be alfalfa, clover, mung bean. Also, keep in a dark place.

5. The greening of alfalfa, clover, buckwheat lettuce or sunflower greens takes place in a sunny window after the sprout gets to growing longer than the seed. The entire process can take 2 days or up to 8-10 days, depending on the individual seed, nut, grain or bean.

Captain Buckwheat Crunch

Soak 3 cups rinsed, hulled buckwheat for 6-7 hours. Rinse 2-3 times daily until a little sprout tail begins to grow. No more than 2-3 days.

Spread out on a solid dehydrator sheet and dehydrate for 2-3 hours at 90 degrees or until dry and crunchy. Store in a covered container in a cupboard. Can use in any sweet nut/seed ball or bar for extra crunch. Can use as cold cereal with nut or seed milk and fresh fruit or as part of a muesli. Can use with any nut or seed sauce. Use to make Crisp Buckwheat Frisbees.

Blanching Almonds

Almonds, when used in pies, cakes, or quantity are sometimes blanched. This can be achieved in two ways: by soaking them overnight or 24 hours, then individually peeling off the skin with your fingers. OR placing the soaked, drained nuts in a bowl and pouring water that has been brought just to a boil over the nuts, leaving the water for about 10 seconds maximum, pouring off, then peeling the skins off easily.

Tip: Be sure to rinse all grains and beans before using or soaking; drain in a colander or strainer and remove any bad beans or seeds or pebbles. Place in a bowl, cover with at least twice as much water and soak as directed.

Twelve Ways to Eat Your Sprouts!

1. Dried: Powdered in drinks, raw soups, patties or whole (buckwheat sprouts) in cereal - they add nutrition and flavor.

2. Drinks: Sunflower seed sprouts, wheat sprouts, mixed sprouts or alfalfa and clover can be juiced or blended into fruit or vegetable juices, smoothies or shakes.

3. Marinated: Marinate garbanzo bean sprouts or soybean sprouts in vinegar, oil, honey and your choice of herbs, then serve as a topping on a green salad. Or marinate buckwheat sprouts in a little tamari sauce, lemon juice, garlic and onion granules. After a couple of hours, drain and dehydrate. Makes a delicious, spicy snack you can eat by the handfuls.

4. Salads: Add alfalfa, clover, sunflower seed or mixed sprouts (lentil-mung-adzuki) to waldorf or fruit salads. Wheat sprouts taste great in fruit salads; cabbage-alfalfa-radish sprouts are great in tossed green salads. Sunflower seeds are great in either fruit or vegetable salads.

5. Seed Cheeses/Yogurts - Sunflower seed sprouts are good for making yogurts and seed cheeses.

6. Sandwich Spreads: Try sunflower seed sprouts mixed with any nut butter.

7. Patties and Loaves: Heap alfalfa or clover sprouts on top of any patty or loaf to add nutrition and flavor.

8. Breads and Crackers: Sprouted wheat, oat groats, sunflower seeds, or rye, are all used to make a dough for a dehydrated bread.

9. Sauces and Dips: Sprouted garbanzo beans make a great hummus.

10. Snacks: Rye, wheat and sunflower seed sprouts mixed with raisins, soaked nuts and/or dates are delicious.

11. Raw Soups: Add fresh sprouts just before serving. Rye sprouts taste like wild rice.

12. Sweets: Wheat, buckwheat (dehydrated) or sunflower seed sprouts are great in nut butter, maple syrup, carob, nut balls. They add flavor, crunch and texture.

Tip: To practice yoga, one needs a flexible body. Cooked foods, salt, dairy products and excessive use of concentrated foods, i.e., nuts, seeds, grains, oil, dried fruit, avocado, sea vegetables, all congest the cells, joints and blood. This can, over time, cause stiffness and aging. Make sure to include juicy fresh fruits and salad greens and juicy vegetables like cucumbers and tomatoes in your daily eating plan.

Breads, Crackers, Cereals

Breads

Sprouted Wheat, Raisin, Cinnamon Bread

2 cups sprouted wheat (Soak 2 cups hard wheatberries overnight, rinse, drain, then
rinse 3 times a day until the sprout is almost as long as the wheat, about 2-3 days.)
Place 2 cups sprouted wheat in food processor.
Add 1 t. cinnamon
Process until very smooth like dough.
Place into bowl and stir in 3/4 cup raisins.
Knead between two sheets plastic wrap.
Form into 3 loaves, flatten to 3/4" high.
Dehydrate on oiled, solid sheet about 8-9 hours, or until crisp on outside and moist but "done" on inside.
Flip loaves and place on mesh tray after first 4 hours.
Tastes great with any nut butter or mashed banana or other fruit spread on top.

Savory Herb Bread

Using 'S' blade of food processor, process the following until a dough-like consistency:
2 1/2 cups sprouted wheat (sprout tails are less than length of wheat berry)
Mix in the remainder ingredients:
1/4 t. each: sage, rosemary, basil, oregano, thyme
1/2 t. Frontier All Purpose Seasoning (dehydrated onion, parsley, lemon peel, basil, thyme, dehydrated garlic, celery, red bell pepper, citric acid, freeze dried whole lemon)
several shakes of sea salt or Herbamare
Continue processing until well-mixed.

If sticky, wrap in plastic wrap and knead. Cut into 3 pieces. Form little loaves or ovals about 3/4" high. Dehydrate on oiled, solid dehydrator sheet - about 4 hours. Remove after 4 hours to a mesh tray to continue dehydrating for about 4 1/2 hours more or until crusty on outside and moist or barely done on inside.

This bread tastes great with mashed avocado spread on it. Slice into very thin slices, or spread over the top of the entire mini-bread loaf.

Chapatis

Sprout 2 cups of wheatberries. Place in food processor and add 1-2 T. olive oil, 1/2 t. sea salt. Process until dough-like. Knead a little and form into long ovals, about 1/8 inch thick. Dehydrate on solid sheet until crisp on outside and still pliable and bendable on inside. Use for open-faced sandwiches. Spread with nut butters and banana slices with raisins or guacamole. Use your imagination. Can fold in half if chapati is pliable.

Crackers

Flax Crackers

2 cups flax seeds, soaked 4-6 hours in 3 cups water
2 T. Bragg's aminos
1 lemon, juiced

Mix all together by spoon in a bowl. Spread thinly on a solid dehydrator sheet. Dehydrate at 105 degrees for 5-6 hours. Flip over onto a mesh tray for 4-5 hours more.

Variations: Add garlic powder and onion powder.
Add chili powder and cumin.
Try Italian seasoning and some sun-dried tomatoes.

Crisp Buckwheat Frisbees

1 cup sprouted buckwheat groats, hulled
1/4 cup olive oil
1 T. soaked raisins
1 garlic clove
1 t. onion granules
1/3 cup carrot pulp (from juicing carrots)
1/3 cup soaked flax seeds

Put all of the above in a food processor and process until very well mixed.

Spoon out onto oiled, solid dehydrator sheets in 6" Frisbee circles, 1/4 inch thick, even from center to edges.

Dehydrate 7-8 hours or until dry enough to be crisp on outside and moister inside. Use as a pizza or bread to spread with your favorite topping.

Cereals

Whole Grain Cereal

1/2 cup sprouted grain (Choose from buckwheat, quinoa, amaranth, millet, wheat, oat groats, barley) Place in bowl. Pour nut milk over grain and slice fresh fruit over cereal. Sprinkle with Five Spice Powder or cinnamon, if desired.

Muesli

1. 1/4-1/2 cup of sprouted, dehydrated buckwheat (Captain Buckwheat Crunch) or sprouted quinoa
2. Pour fresh yogurt or fruity sauce over sprouts.
3. Add sliced bananas and a few sprouted sun seeds and chopped almonds.
4. Top with soaked, dried cherries, apricots, dates, fresh chopped apples, figs, prunes.
5. Garnish with cinnamon, Five Spice Powder, mace, or nutmeg.

Grape Nutty Cereal

In a food processor, process equal parts sprouted wheat and raisins. Knead the 'dough' well, spread 1/4" high on solid dehydrator sheet and dehydrate until very dry and crisp. Crumble into granola-like clumps and store in covered container. Use to sprinkle on salads, as cold cereal, or to sprinkle on fruit or seed yogurt.

Blueberry Breakfast

Spoon Cream in bottom of bowl. Add washed,drained blueberries. Sprinkle a little Captain Buckwheat Crunch on top. **Cream**: Mash two bananas with a grated apple, 1 t. maple syrup or honey, some chopped nuts, 1 teaspoon of lemon juice and a sprinkle of shredded, unsweetened coconut.

Chart for Seeds/Beans/Grains

Sprout	Container	Amount	Soak	Days to Sprout	Length of Sprout	Sunlight?
Seeds						
Alfalfa	jar/basket	3 T.	5 hrs.	3-6 days	1-3 inches	after 2 days
Broccoli	jar/basket	2 T.	8 hrs.	3-4 days	1-2 inches	after 2-3 days
Cabbage	jar/basket	1 T.	6 hrs.	4-5 days	1-2 inches	after 2-3 days
Flax	jar	see recipe	see recipe	won't sprout	O	
Radish	jar/basket	3 T.	6 hours	3-5 days	1/2 inch to 2 inches	after 2-3 days
Red Clover	jar/basket	3 T.	6 hours	4-6 days	1-3 inches	
Sesame, hulled	jar	see recipe	8 hours	won't sprout		
Sunflower, hulled	jar	see recipe	8 hours	1-2 days	less than length of seed	no
Grains						
Amaranth	jar	see recipe	3-5 hours	2-3 days	0 to 1/4 inch	no
Barley (hulless)	jar	see recipe	6 hours	1/2 to 1 day	0 to 1/4 inch	no
Buckwheat Groats	jar	see recipe	6 hours max	1-2 days	1/4 to 1/2 inch	no
Oat Groats	jar	see recipe	8 hours	1-2 days	0	no
Quinoa (rinsewell)	jar	see recipe	3 4 hours	2-3 days	0 to 1/2 inch	no
Rye	jar	see recipe	6-8 hours	2-3 days	1/4 to 1/2 inch	no
Spelt	jar	see recipe	6 hours	1-2 days	9 to 1/4 inch	no
Hard Wheat	jar	see recipe	8-10 hours	2-3 days	less than length of seed	no
Soft Wheat	jar	see recipe	8-10 hours	2 days	half as long as seed	no

Sprout	Container	Amount	Soak	Days to Sprout	Length of Sprout	Sunlight?
<u>Beans</u>						
Adzuki	jar	1/4 cup	12 hours	3-5 days	1/2 to 1 inch	no
Chickpea (Garbanzo)	jar	see recipe	12-48 hours	2-4 days	1/4 to 1 inch	no
Mung	jar	see recipe	8 hours	2-6 days	1/2 to 4 inches	no
Lentil	jar	1/4 cup	8 hours	2-3 days	1/4 to 1 inch	no
Soybeans	jar	see recipe	12-24 hours	2-3 days max.	1/4 to 1/2 inch	no
<u>Nuts</u>						
Almonds	jar	see recipe	8-10 hours	1-2 days, or soaked only	0 to 1/8 inch	
Cashews, rinse well	jar	see recipe	6 hours	soaked only		
Filberts	jar	see recipe	6 hours	soaked only		
Pecans	jar	see recipe	6 hours or less	soaked only		
Walnuts	jar	see recipe	6 hours or less	soaked only		
Pine Nuts	jar	see recipe	6 hours or less	soaked only		
<u>Greens/Lettuce</u>			**In jar/water**	**Harvest Time**		
Buckwheat, unhulled	tray w/soil	2 cups/tray	8-10 hours	7-9 days	4-6 inches	after 3 days/cvrd
Sunflower, unhulled	tray w/soil	2 cups/tray	8-10 hours	5-8 days	4-6 inches	after 3 days/cvrd
Wheatberries, hard (for wheat grass)	tray w/soil	2 cups/tray	8-12 hours	8-10 days	4-8 inches	after 3 days/cvrd

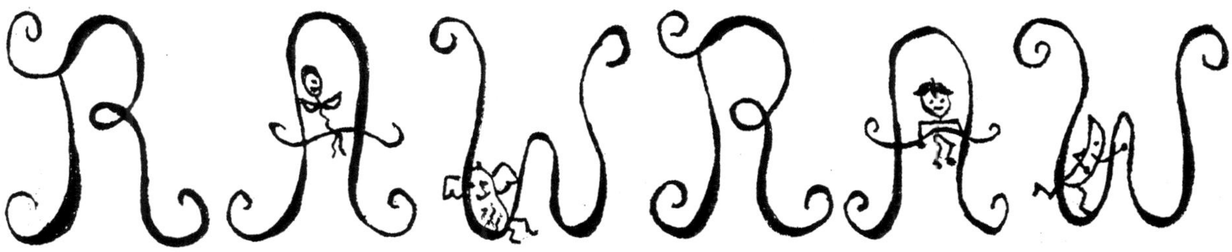

CHAPTER V
SNACKS
SWEET, SPICY, FROZEN, ON-THE-GO

Sweet Snacks

South of the Border Bananas

Cut peeled bananas into thirds. Dip in fresh pineapple juice and roll in unsweetened, shredded, coconut, ground sunflower seeds or Almond-Cinnamon Mixture.

Funny Faces

Use flat sprouted bread, Buckwheat Frisbees, Wheat Chapatis or a round melon or apple slice.

Spread with a nut butter. Make a face using sprouts or carrot curls for hair, radish slivers or apple slice for mouth, cherry tomato or strawberry for nose, almonds for eyes, olive slivers for eyebrows. Kids can make their own individual open-faced snack.

Tip: Freeze whole grapes, red and green, for a tasty, summertime snack. Pit cherries and freeze whole. They can be chewed or sucked. Try dehydrating these same fruits. Cut each in half or dry whole until chewy.

Fresh Applesauce with Cinnamon

2-3 apples, washed, unpeeled, chopped
1/4 cup raisins
1/4 cup apple juice or orange juice
1-2 T. lemon juice or orange juice
1 t. cinnamon

Blend raisins with apple or orange juice.

Add raisin mixture to chopped apples and cinnamon. and blend until of applesauce consistency. Serve immediately.

Variation: Omit the cinnamon and sprinkle it on when blended apples are in a bowl.

Layered Parfait Dessert

In parfait glasses, layer the following ingredients: sweet yogurt, sliced bananas, a few sunflower seeds or sunflower seed sprouts, yogurt, sliced strawberries, chopped, soaked almonds, yogurt, kiwi slices. Continue layering, ending with fruit or yogurt and topped with a few chopped nuts and a sprinkle of 5 Spice Powder.

Fruit Kebobs

Use chunks of papaya, pineapple, grapes, cherries, mangoes, bananas, peaches, apricots, oranges, and/or kiwi. String a variety onto bamboo skewers. Arrange on a platter, in a fan-shape or as spokes in a wheel/mandala pattern. Drizzle with lime or orange juice.

Refrigerate, covered. Just before serving, drizzle Ambrosia Dressing over all or place sauce in small, individual bowls for dipping.

Spicy Snacks

Spicy Captain Buckwheat Crunch

Soak 3 cups rinsed, hulled buckwheat for 6-7 hours. Rinse 2-3 times daily until a little sprout tail begins to grow. No more than 2-3 days.

Soak sprouted buckwheat in lemon juice, tamari sauce, garlic and onion powder (to cover the sprouts) for an hour. Drain and dehydrate on a solid dehydrator sheet for 2-3 hours or until dry and crunchy. Keep in covered container and eat by the handfuls or sprinkle on top of your salad for a tasty crunch.

Crisp Buckwheat Frisbees

1 cup sprouted buckwheat groats
1/4 cup olive oil
1 T. soaked raisins
1 garlic clove
1 t. onion granules
1/3 cup carrot pulp (from juicing carrots)
1/3 cup soaked flax seeds

Put all of the above in a food processor and process until very well mixed.

Spoon out onto oiled solid dehydrator sheets in 6" Frisbee circles, 1/4 inch thick, evenly from center to edges.

Dehydrate 7-8 hours or until dry enough to transfer to a mesh tray. Dehydrate another 7-8 hours.

Crust should be very dry, no moisture or soft insides. Will store in a loosely covered container in a dry place for a couple of weeks if very dry.

Great as a pizza crust, with pesto, tomato puree (from sun-dried tomatoes), or olive oil spread on crust, topped with raw veggies. Also great with mashed avocado spread on top, with paprika or alfalfa sprouts. Tuna-4-2 spreads very nicely on top of a crust.

Spicy Jicama 'Stix'

1 small jicama

Peel and slice into sticks the size of French fries.

Place in a shallow glass bowl. Drizzle a little olive oil over 'stix' and mix well.

Sprinkle a mixture of chili powder, paprika, herbal seasoning or sea salt over the 'stix'. Stir well.

Place on a small plate beside a green salad and enjoy the crispy, spicy 'stix'.

Variation: For a delicious, sweet taste, drizzle lime juice from one lime over jicama 'stix'. Stir well. Sprinkle a mixture of onion powder and paprika over the 'stix' and mix well. Serve on a plate of greens with lime wedges. This is my favorite - I usually place them beside my salad.

Variation: For a quick, crunchy protein snack, place jicama 'stix' on a plate with a small bowl of your favorite nut butter in the center. Dip 'stix' into nut butter as you eat them. Can use guacamole in place of nut butter.

Mushroom Caps

Select shitake, portobello or white or brown mushrooms. Remove stems. Pour a mixture of the following over the mushrooms and stir to coat evenly. Marinate in refrigerator for at least an hour:

1 lemon, juiced
2-3 T. olive oil
1 T. tamari sauce
1/8 t. garlic granules

Drain off marinade. Spoon any seed sauce into caps (mushrooms turned upside down). Sprinkle paprika over sauce and add a sprig of parsley.

Wholly Guacamole!

Spread a chapati or Buckwheat Frisbee with your favorite miso dressing. Spread guacamole all over it. Heap with alfalfa sprouts, grated carrots and sprouted sunflower seeds, grated radish and zucchini. Add a tomato slice or two, dollop with Hearty Party Dip and enjoy.

Easy 'Cup' Snacks

red, yellow or green peppers (seeds and top removed)
tomatoes (hollowed out)
cucumbers or zucchini, (cut in half lengthwise and hollowed out)

Blend inside pulp (if tomato, cucumber or zucchini) with sunflower seeds to make a thick sauce. Refill tomato, peppers, cucumbers or zucchini and serve with parsley on top or on a bed of alfalfa sprouts.

Variation: Fill green or red pepper or tomato with Quinoa Tabouleh.

Tip: When there is an abundance of garden-fresh vegetables, chop or slice and dehydrate for chips or later use in seed yogurts and cheese or sauces and dips.

Chips Ahoy!

Yam Chips - Scrub yam. Peel and slice thin. Dehydrate 3-6 hours or until desired crispness. Can be chewy or crisp. Halfway through dehydrating, sprinkle onion powder or kelp, if desired.

Zucchini Chips - Scrub zucchinis. Slice thin. Dehydrate 3-6 hours or until desired crispness. Can be chewy or crisp. Halfway through dehydrating, sprinkle onion powder or dried basil or oregano on them, if desired.

Other Chips: Dehydrate thin slices of cucumber, parsnips and eggplant. Use as chips for dipping into sauces and dips.

More Chips for Dips

green crackers, flax crackers, corn crackers, oat crackers, etc. (all dehydrated)
dried zucchini, Jerusalem artichokes, yams - all thinly sliced

Also try apple wedges, carrot sticks, celery sticks
sliced jicama, cherry tomatoes, thin slices of turnips, beets and rutabagas
cauliflowerets, broccoli flowers, thinly sliced broccoli stalks
cucumber sticks, carrot circles
sliced mushrooms
green onions, green, red, and yellow bell pepper strips

Tip: Raw carrot, celery and yam can be sliced thinly into chips, placed in a jar filled with lemon water and refrigerated overnight. Then drain and use as chips for dipping.

Frozen Snacks

Jawbreakers

For individual jawbreakers, freeze red or green grapes, sweet cherries, watermelon and cantaloupe balls. To eat, chew or suck on frozen fruit very carefully. They are delicious and make a great snack. Store in a covered container in your freezer.

Carob-Banana Pops

Cut bananas in half, insert a popsicle stick in one end and freeze on cookie sheets until firm. Then dip in a thickened carob sauce, roll in ground Almond-Cinnamon Mixture or ground walnuts. Individually wrap in plastic wrap and place in freezer. Eat as a popsicle.

Carob Sauce

Use raw carob powder, maple syrup, olive oil, vanilla extract. Add enough carob powder to make fairly thick.

Snow Cones

Using a hand-cranked snow cone machine, place cubes of fresh, frozen orange juice, pink grapefruit juice, or frozen fruit puree (peach, strawberry, plum). It will 'shave' the ice until you have a lovely snow cone.

Variation: Shave ice cubes until you have a snow cone, then pour grape juice or cherry juice over for a delicious snow cone.

Popsicles

Freeze any fruit puree or combination of fruit purees or juices in paper cups with a popsicle stick placed in the center. Freeze until firm, then peel off cups for a tasty treat.

Snacks for On-the-Go

Gummy Bugs

For fun gummy bugs, dehydrate slices of fresh strawberries, grape slices, kiwi half-circles, and cherries until chewy. Can take on trips and chew when bored.

Pick-Me-Ups

Whenever you are hungry for a mid-morning or mid-afternoon snack, try the following raw foods:

an apple
kiwi fruit - peeled and sliced
one-half a banana
ruby red grapefruit
a handful of mixed, raw nuts (Brazil, walnuts, pecans, almonds, cashews
raw or sprouted sunflower seeds)
a glass of freshly juiced carrot juice
an orange
raw almond butter on a piece of sprouted, dehydrated bread (made from wheat, kamut or spelt)
a few baby carrots or cucumber slices with raw Oregon Hummus as a dip
same as above with Party Pate' or Hearty Party Dip.
a nut butter, coconut-seed-nut-dried fruit-energy bar of your own concoction

Tip: Always keep a soft cooler or lunch bag with a frozen ice pack to keep your snacks in. Many snacks do not require refrigeration. In the case of nuts and seeds, just put them in a zip-lock bag and keep in your purse or car.

My first crisis didn't occur until Week 3, Day 2. I had gone to the gym, then immediately to the store to pick up the ingredients for a punch that I was making for a wedding. I showered, took time for my Power Smoothie, dashed off to the wedding, then helped at the reception. All around me were people eating wrapped chocolate heart candy, wedding cake and drinking punch. I had brought some High Protein Sesame Seed Energy Bars for people to eat. By the time I got to the tray there were only 2 remaining. I took one and a few sips of frozen orange juice concentrate, reconstituted (still live and uncooked). After the wedding reception I went to a movie and had nothing, then to my son's home to give him some presents. They were eating, but nothing that I could eat. I went to the store to pick up a grapefruit, then home. I was so famished, having rushed all day, being so active. I thought, I'm too tired to prepare anything; I'll just eat this grapefruit. But I opened the refrigerator and there were all the salad fixings, washed and ready to be put into a salad bowl. I decided to make a Super Sushi Roll and a little salad. It was worth the effort. So I highly recommend that if you don't know how long it will be before you can eat, take some nuts and seeds for a little protein, and maybe an energy ball or a piece of fruit. Packed in a lunchbox with a frozen ice pack, most anything will stay cool and fresh all day.

Stuffed Snacks

Stuff dates, celery or apple halves with any of the following:

1. a whole almond, walnut or pecan (Slit the date and insert nut half and close)
2. a mixture of 2 T. orange juice, 2 T. sunflower seed sprouts, 2 T. sweet yogurt
3. seed cheese mixed with grated carrots and raisins
4. seed cheese or yogurt mixed with chopped cucumber and minced onion, celery and radish
5. nut butter with raisins and sunflower seed sprouts

Cup O' Crunch

Mix raw almonds, cashews, pecans, walnuts, sunflower seeds, pumpkin seeds. Soak briefly with tamari sauce mixed with a little garlic and onion granules. Drain and dehydrate until dry. Store in covered container.

Banana Burrito!

On a Romaine lettuce leaf, place one whole, peeled banana. Spread your favorite nut butter on top of the banana. Sprinkle some raisins and sunflower seeds or sunflower seed sprouts over all and roll up banana and leaf until you have a nice, leafy green burrito. Great as a snack or for lunch. Easy to pack in a lunch pail with an ice pack.

Tooty Fruity Burrito!

On a red leaf lettuce leaf, gently dollop some mashed, ripe fruit (peaches, strawberries, apples); sprinkle with nutmeg, anise, cinnamon and sunflower seed sprouts or chopped nuts. Roll up around filling and eat.

Stuffed Apple Lunch

Cut the top off an apple and scoop out the core and some of the apple, leaving a cavity to fill. Make a mixture of chopped raw nuts, sunflower seed sprouts, grated apple and a little nut butter. Spoon into hole, place the top of apple back on and wrap in plastic wrap to hold it together. Great for school or work lunch. Take on hikes or car trips.

Live Foods Trail Mix

Mix raw nuts (at least 3 kinds) sunflower seeds, raisins, Captain Buckwheat Crunch, shredded, unsweetened coconut and dried fruit (at least 3 kinds). Pack in zip-lock bags.

Hiking Energy Trail Balls

In food processor, using 'S' blade, chop the following:

1/4 cup pumpkin seeds
1/4 cup walnuts
1/4 cup almonds
1/4 cup cashews
1/4 cup sunflower seeds
1/4 cup raisins

Stir in:

1/4 cup raw almond butter or tahini (Begin with 1/4 cup nut butter. Add more as needed to hold nuts and seeds together.)
1/4 cup Captain Buckwheat Crunch
2 T. maple syrup
1 T. honey
1-2 T. Green Protein powder

Roll in a log and chill. Slice or break off roll and roll into balls.

Sprouts, Raisins and Dates

Toss 1/2 cup wheat sprouts, sunflower seed sprouts, Captain Buckwheat Crunch, 1/2 cup raisins, 2 chopped dates and 1/2 t. cinnamon. Refrigerate and mix well before eating.

Dried Fruit Roll-ups

Blend any of the following combinations in a blender, pour onto plastic wrap or solid dehydrator sheet and dehydrate until bendable and chewy. Roll up in plastic wrap and store in covered container.

Apple Pie: 2 c. apple puree, 2 T. lemon juice, 1 t. cinnamon, dash nutmeg, dash cloves
Cherry: 1 c. apple puree and 1 cup cherry puree, 2 T. lemon juice, 1/2 t. anise seed (ground)
Pear: 2 c. pear puree, 1 T. lemon juice, 1/2 t. cinnamon
Banana: 2 c. banana puree, 2 T. lemon juice

Barb's Sweet Sugar Plums

2 cups whole almonds
1/4 cup honey
2 teaspoons grated orange zest
1 1/2 teaspoons cinnamon
1/2 teaspoon allspice
1/2 teaspoon nutmeg
1 cup finely chopped dried apricots
1 cup finely chopped pitted dates
1 cup blender-powdered coconut, almond or cashews (a fine powder)

Combine honey, orange zest and spices in medium bowl. Add almonds, dates and apricots and mix well,

Pinch off rounded teaspoon-sized pieces and roll into balls. (Rinse your hands often, as mixture is very sticky). Roll balls in finely powdered almond meal, cashew meal or dried, unsweetened coconut powder and refrigerate in single layers between sheets of waxed paper in airtight container for up to one month.

Their flavor improves after ripening for several days.

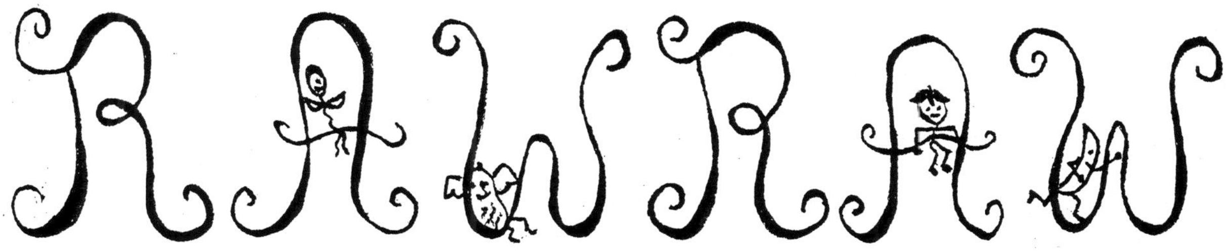

CHAPTER VI
FOOD PROCESSOR MAGIC
(SAUCES, DIPS-SPREADS, BUTTERS SALSAS, YOGURTS, SEED CHEESES)

Sauces/Dips-Spreads/ Butters

Sauces

Seed Sauce

1/2 cup tahini
1/2 lime, juiced
a little water
herbal seasoning

Cream.

Variation: Use pecan meal or sunflower seed or almond meal with water in place of tahini.

Sunrise Sauce

In food processor, using the 'S' blade, grind
1/2 cup sunflower seeds, soaked
1/2 cup pine nuts, soaked
1/4 cup almonds, soaked
Add:
1 seeded, red bell pepper
1/2 lemon, juiced
1 clove garlic, chopped (optional)
1 rounded T. nutritional yeast
1-2 t. tamari sauce

Sauce should be fairly smooth with small bits of nuts and pepper. Spoon into a bowl and use as a dip for raw vegetables. Spoon over top of green salads or mix into Broccoli-in-Bed. Spread a little bit on your favorite patty. Store covered in refrigerator. Will keep up to 5 days. This sauce can be spread thin on a solid dehydrator sheet
and dehydrated until very dry. Break into pieces and place into a sandwich baggie. Crumble with a rolling pin or glass and store in a large bottle in refrigerator. Shake over salads for a unique "cheesy" taste. Its pink color looks like a pimiento cream cheese.

Variation: Substitute onion powder for garlic, and chopped cucumber or juicy tomatoes for the red pepper.

Pecan Sauce

2 cups pecans, soaked 1 hour
2 cups water
1/4 sweet onion
2 t. poultry seasoning
1 T. olive oil
tamari sauce or Herbamare, to taste

Blend until like a gravy. Serve over Cauliflower Mash or any veggie loaf or patty.

Mushroom Sauce

Blend the following ingredients in a blender until smooth:

1/4 cup water
3 T. olive oil
1 clove garlic
1 green onion - include tops
dash kelp
1/4 cup fresh, button mushrooms
1/4 cup packed parsley (stems cut)
1-2 t. tamari sauce
dash cayenne

Spoon over Cauliflower Mash with fresh, chopped white mushrooms or rehydrated shitake mushrooms on top. Use as a sauce or gravy for any patty or loaf.

'Hot Tamale' Sauce

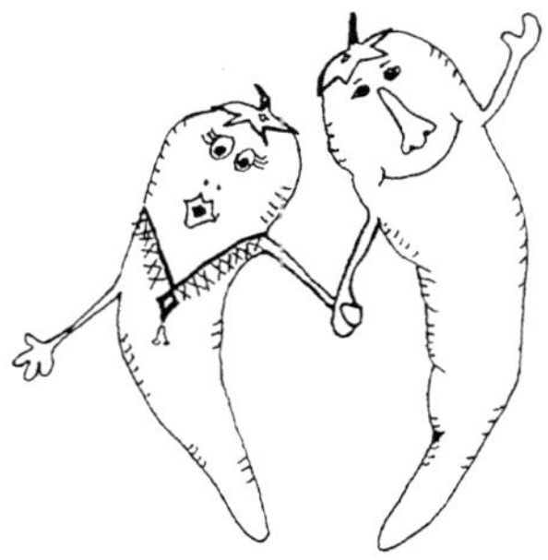

Blend the following ingredients in a blender until smooth:

1/4 cup olive oil
1/2 - 1" slice of jalapeno pepper (seeded)
1 t. tamari sauce or aminos
1 clove garlic
fresh or dried basil (always use twice as much fresh as dried)
2-3 T. sweet onion
1 sprig parsley
1 t. paprika

Pour over baby leaf spinach and other greens and top with grated carrot or beet.

Variation: Can add chopped green veggies and mushrooms.

Pizza Sauce

Blend in a blender until smooth:

1 cup sun-dried tomatoes, soaked
1/2 cup fresh tomatoes, diced
1 T. apple cider vinegar
1 T. maple syrup
1 clove garlic
1/4 cup fresh, chopped basil
2 T. olive oil
Veg-It or Herbamare or All Purpose Seasoning to taste

Spread on Crisp Buckwheat Frisbees or Chapatis. Delicious!

Spinach Pesto

In a food processor, using 'S' blade, process:

1 bunch spinach
a few sprigs of parsley
some olive oil
sea salt to taste

Mix in and add to taste:

1 T. lemon juice
1 clove garlic, minced
1-2 T. slivered almonds (or soaked, peeled, sliced almonds)

Basil Pesto

In a food processor, using 'S' blade, process:

3 cups fresh basil
1/2 cup sunflower seeds, soaked overnight, then rinsed
2 T. lemon juice
2 cloves garlic, minced
1 t. All-Purpose Seasoning

Stir in by hand:

1 tomato, diced

Variation: Replace sunflower seeds with same amount of soaked pine nuts. Great spread on dehydrated crackers or Crisp Buckwheat Frisbees.

Sprouted Sunflower Seed Sauce

Blend all but the water in a blender until smooth:

1 1/4 cups sprouted sunflower seeds
2 cloves garlic
1/4 cup lemon juice or more to taste
2 T. Bragg's aminos
dash cayenne, dash of kelp

When blended, add water, a little at a time, up to a cup until of desired consistency. If using to stuff Super Sushi Rolls, red bell peppers or cabbage leaves, use less water; if using as a sauce on veggies, salads, patties or loaves, use a little more water.

Fruity Seed Sauce

Blend all in a blender until smooth and creamy:
1 cup orange juice
2-3 T. soaked seeds or nuts
1 T. lemon juice
water, as needed

Dips-Spreads

For spreading on Buckwheat Frisbees, crackers, zucchini chips, sliced zucchini or cucumbers, lettuce leaves, etc. Some dips and spreads are great for fruit slices to be dipped into. Some are great as fillings or stuffings.

Hearty Party Dip

1 1/2 cups sunflower seeds – Soak overnight and sprout for 1 day.
1 t. flax seeds, ground
1/2 t. curry powder
1/3 cup lemon juice
1/2 cup chopped parsley
1 t. tamari sauce
1 T. Bragg's liquid aminos
2 T. chopped, red onion
1 garlic clove (opt.)

Put all in food processor and blend until smooth. Spoon into bowl and add 1/3 cup diced sweet red pepper.

Store covered in refrigerator. Makes a great dip for carrot and cucumber sticks or slices, broccoli and cauliflower. Can be used as a filling for Super Sushi Rolls and can be spooned into a hollowed-out red bell pepper and topped with sunflower seeds and alfalfa sprouts.

Green, Creamy Dip

Cream 1 avocado with 1 cucumber and 3 T. lime juice. Serve in a bowl with thin cucumber slices to dip.

Oregon Hummus

2 cups sprouted chickpeas (garbanzo beans)
1/4 cup lemon juice
3-4 T. raw tahini
1/4 cup parsley, loosely packed
2 garlic cloves, chopped
1/4 t. cumin
1/4 t. cayenne pepper

Process the above. Should be thick. Gradually add olive oil to make smooth and creamy, yet still thick. (approx. 1/4 cup, but more is okay, too)

Serve as a side dish when having a salad. Makes a great dip for carrot sticks, cauliflower, jicama, cucumber slices. Slice cucumber diagonally into ovals and spread a little hummus on each. Top with a sprig of parsley and sprinkle with paprika, for a great snack.

Cauliflower Mash (White or Green)

2 1/2 cups cauliflower, cut into small flowerets (include part of the stalk on each one)
1/4 cup lemon juice

Blend the above in the blender until very smooth.

Add all the rest below and blend until smooth.

1/2 cup raw cashews
1 T. herbal seasoning
1/2 t. garlic granules
1 t. onion powder or granules
1 t. Dr. Bragg's aminos
1 T. olive oil

Use a spatula to transfer to a bowl. When ready to serve, place a dollop on a red lettuce leaf. Sprinkle with paprika, garnish with a sprig of parsley and make a well in the center for 1 t. flax oil. This has the look and mouth-feel of mashed potatoes, and surprisingly, tastes very similar.

You can also use it as a dip for carrot sticks, as a spread on crackers, or on Crispy Buckwheat Frisbees.

Variation: For Green Cauliflower Mash - add 2-3 T. chopped parsley

Party Paté

In a small bowl, stir the following and let set for 5 minutes:

1 1/2 t. agar agar flakes (a seaweed used like gelatin) Could use a little psyllium powder or ground flax seed

1 T. cold water

After 5 minutes add 2 T. very warm water, mix well and let stand another 5 minutes.

In food processor, using grater attachment, process:

3 mini snack carrots

1 1/2 cups raw cashew pieces

Empty food processor. Change grater attachment to 'S' blade.

Add cashews, carrots, agar agar back to processor bowl.

Add remaining ingredients. Process until very smooth.

1/2 cup sprouted sunflower seeds

2 T. nutritional yeast

2 T. lemon juice

1 T. olive oil

1/4 t. Veg-It

1/2 t. All Purpose Seasoning

1/4 t. onion granules

1/8 t. cayenne pepper

When very smooth, spoon into oiled mold, like a small plastic take-home tray. Cover with plastic wrap and refrigerate overnight. When ready to use, place on serving plate with some greens and tip over and squeeze sides of mold to remove. Slice thin with a butter knife (about 1/4" thick) and spread on crackers or cucumber slices. Sprinkle paprika over all.

Variation: Add 4-6 olives along with rest of ingredients. When ready to serve, lay some olive slices on top of paté and garnish with a sprig of parsley.

Tip: These sauces, dips and pates can be used in many ways. Some make great salad dressings on top of a salad. Some can be a dip for veggies and dehydrated crackers or chips. They make great fillings for Super Sushi Rolls and lettuce burritos, as well as stuffing a red bell pepper or zucchini boat.

Sprouted Sunflower Seed Dip

In food processor, using 'S' blade, process until smooth:

1 cup sunflower seeds, sprouted 2 days or just until nub of sprout appears
3 T. red onion, chopped
1 T. lemon juice
2 T. tahini
1 t. white miso
1/4" slice ginger root
1 clove garlic
2-3 T. water (as needed)
1/2" slice jalapeno pepper, seeded

Mix in by hand the following:

1 cup finely grated carrot. Transfer all to a bowl and refrigerate. Use as a filling for Super Sushi Rolls, lettuce or cabbage roll-ups or as a dip for raw veggies.

Nut & Seed Butters

Finely grind nuts or seeds in a blender or nut grinder until powdered. If using a nut grinder, transfer to a blender. Add 1 t. of olive or flax oil per cup of nuts to make a smooth, nut butter. Try processing in a food processor. Choose from almond, walnuts, cashews, sesame seeds (unbleached, hulled), sunflower seeds, macadamia nuts. Refrigerate in a covered container to prevent rancidity. Sesame butter is tahini, which is rich in calcium, protein and unsaturated fatty acids.

Nut Butter With . . .

1. Nut butter and orange juice - Mix 1 t. orange juice into a nut butter, add a few raisins for a cracker or bread spread.
2. Grate some apple, raw yam, add cinnamon and finely chopped nuts. Mix in a little nut butter until spreadable onto a chapati or sprouted wheat bread.
3. Stir in a little water with 2-3 T. almond butter. Spread over sliced banana chunks.
4. Mix a little nut butter into grated carrot and a few raisins for a tasty spread.
5. Heap alfalfa sprouts onto a nut butter spread on a chapati or sprouted grain bread (Crisp Buckwheat Frisbees).

Tahini Spread

Mix together 1/4 cup tahini and 2 T. almond or cashew butter. Add 1/4 cup finely chopped nuts. Refrigerate. Use on crackers, breads or on lettuce for a lettuce burrito.

Tahini Topping

Mix 1/3 cup raw tahini, 2 T. honey or maple syrup, 1/2 t. cinnamon, 2 T. apple or orange juice. Chill in refrigerator, covered. Use as a topping or dip for fruit or spread on a sweet bread and top with grated apples.

Peach Lover's Delight

Spread your favorite raw nut/seed butter on sprouted wheat or other grain bread. Slice fresh peaches on top.

Monkey Mash

Mash 1 ripe banana into 1/4 to 1/2 cup nut butter, 1/2 t. cinnamon, a handful of raisins OR dates, and 1-2 t. of shredded coconut. Spread on apple slices or on dehydrated sprouted bread or crackers.

'Cheese', Sprouts and Nut Butter

Mix nut butter, a seed cheese and sunflower seed sprouts together and use as a spread or dip.

Avocado Butter

Place 2 large avocados in blender with juice of 1/2 lemon. Add a dash of cayenne pepper and herbs of your choice. Blend until creamy, then use on sprouted breads or crackers. Can be prepared in a bowl using a fork to mash.

'We Love Your Body' Guacamole

3-4 avocados, mashed or diced (your preference)
4 fresh tomatoes, diced
1 medium onion, chopped fine or
2 green onions, thinly sliced
1/2 t. garlic granules
1/4 t. chili powder
1/2 jalapeño pepper, minced
1 small bunch chopped cilantro
1 lime, juiced

Mix together in bowl by stirring.

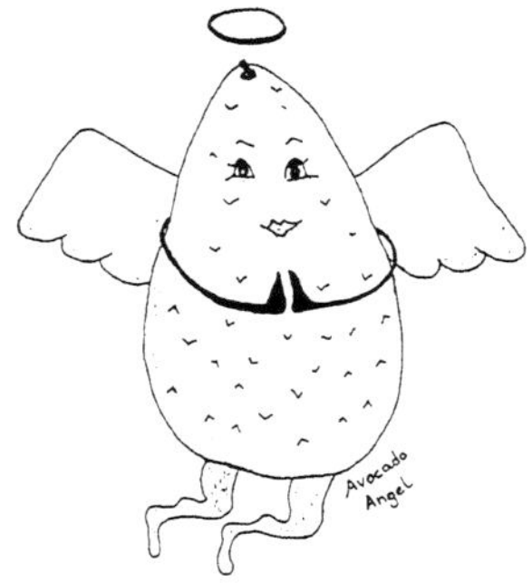

Green Goddess Better Butter

Blend until pureed in a food processor or blender:

3/4 cup loosely packed cilantro leaves, rinsed and drained
1/2 cup raw cashews
1/2 lime, juiced
3 T. olive oil
1 garlic clove
1/4" slice of ginger, peeled
1/2 t. All Purpose Seasoning

Place into a covered container and refrigerate until ready to use. Great as an accompaniment to a green salad or shredded veggies.

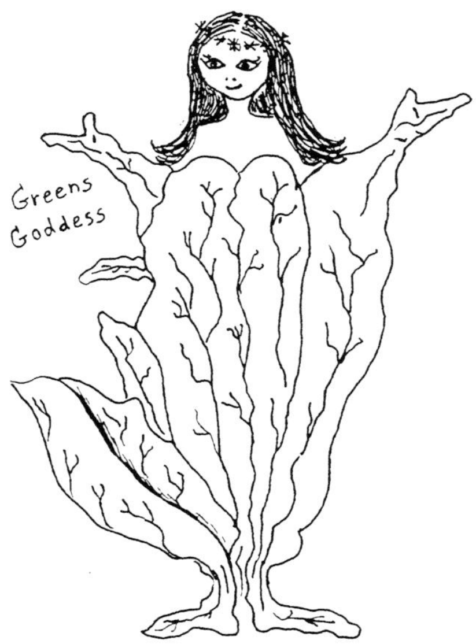

Salsas

Pineapple Salsa

2 cups diced, fresh pineapple
1 diced sweet onion (Walla Walla)
1/2 finely chopped jalapeño pepper
1 small bunch cilantro, stems removed
1/2 lime, juiced
sea salt and/or cayenne to taste

Mix all together in a bowl. Chill.

WLYB Salsa

2-3 fresh, diced tomatoes
1 diced, medium onion
1/4 cup fresh, chopped parsley
2 minced garlic cloves
1/2 t. sea salt/kelp mixture
dash of cayenne pepper
1/8 t. ground cumin
1/8 t. chili powder
1 t. olive oil

Combine ingredients in a bowl. Refrigerate until well-chilled.

Cheryl's Tropical Salsa

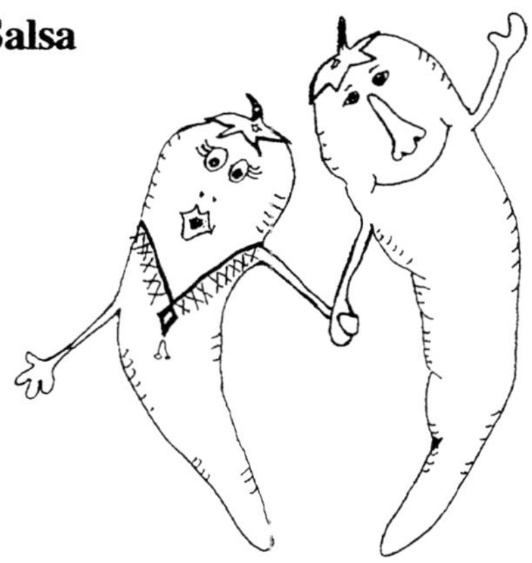

1 ripe papaya, peeled, seeded and chopped
1/2 cup chopped, red onion
1/4 cup chopped, fresh cilantro
2 T. fresh lime juice
1/2 t. grated lime peel
1/2 t. sea salt (optional)
1/2 jalapeño pepper, seeded, sliced and minced

Combine all ingredients in a bowl.

Variations: use nectarines or mango in place of papaya
use lemon juice in place of lime

Green Salsa Challenge

At my local farmer's market I discovered a fresh, spicy, green salsa, uncooked, organic and delicious. The only ingredient I objected to was the xanthan gum. I figured I could add a little agar-agar flakes (similar to gelatin but is a sea vegetable) to the water to help thicken the salsa, or a teaspoon or less of psyllium powder or ground flax seed to thicken. The following were the ingredients listed on the container, written from most to least:

Ingredients: tomatillos, water, onions, apple cider vinegar, garlic, jalapeno peppers, cilantro, salt, cumin, xanthan gum 14 fluid ounces (This salsa is slightly chunky, and not very thick. The xanthan gum seems to be the binding holding it together.)

My challenge to you is to experiment and come up with something that matches your taste buds--hot and sassy, if that's what you like, or mellowed down without the fire. Go for it. You can even substitute an ingredient and add something you prefer, if you like. I don't create a recipe totally from scratch. I use previous experience, intuition, tasting as I create, knowing what fruits go together for best digestion, what veggies make tasty, colorful combinations, etc.

If it's something totally strange, I look at recipes and add or subtract what I want according to what I have at hand or what I do or do not like. Then I prepare it, tweaking it each time I make it until it has just the right spices or herbs, just the best texture, or eye-appeal to it. Taste, it goes without saying, is foremost. So, take these salsa ingredients and make them into something of your very own creation. I spoon this liberally over my salad greens for a great flavor. There are virtually no calories (12 per 2 T.), zero fat, zero carbs, and zero protein.

My experimental concoction can be found at the end of this chapter. Don't cheat and look. Try your own. That way, when you know you should throw out your favorite salad dressing, for example, write down the ingredients first, in the order listed (from most to least), then experiment and try to duplicate a healthier and tastier raw, uncooked version. It's okay to leave out an egg, or mayonnaise. You can substitute or just leave out.

Here are the ingredients listed on my husband's favorite French Dressing (a name brand):
Ingredients: water, corn syrup, sugar, vinegar, modified food starch, salt, contains less than 2% of tomato paste, xanthan gum, garlic juice, with potassium sorbate and calcium disodium EDTA as preservatives, propylene glycol alginate, mustard flour, paprika, artificial color, yellow #6, vitamin E acetate

2 T. contains 11 grams of Carbohydrates, 0 grams Fat, 0 grams Protein, 5 grams sugar, 300 mg. Sodium

I know one can make a healthier, and tastier version of French Dressing. For sure, omit the preservatives, the sugar, corn syrup, the propylene glycol alginate and the artificial color. Try paprika or red bell pepper for color.

High C Salsa

3 oranges, peeled, with segments cut into fourths
1 red grapefruit, peeled, with segments cut into fourths
1 jalapeno, minced
1 small red onion, diced
1/4 cup packed, chopped cilantro
sea salt to taste
a little orange juice from one segment

Mix all together in a bowl. Cover and chill.

Yogurts

Cinn-fully Delicious Yogurt

1/2 cup sprouted sunflower seeds
3/4 cup raw cashews
Grind the above in a food processor.
Add: 1 cup fresh orange juice. Blend with nuts and seeds. Add 1/2 cup more orange juice, 1/2 t. white miso, 1 t. cinnamon, 1/3 cup pitted dates.

Pour into a jar, cover with cheesecloth held by a rubber band and place at room temperature or slightly warmer for 3 hours. Pour off any whey. Eat as is or dip apple slices or jicama 'stix' into yogurt.

Variation: Yogurt can be made into a cheese if jar is placed upside down over a rack with a bowl to catch the "whey". Do this in the refrigerator until no more dripping occurs. Use as a "cheese" spread.

Variation: Squeeze half of a lime over a bowl of jicama 'stix'. Then sprinkle cinnamon over all. Arrange like spokes of a wheel on a plate with a dollop of yogurt in the center. Dip the 'stix' into the yogurt for a nutritious snack.

Fresh Fruity Yogurt

In blender blend the following:

1/2 cup Sunflower Seed Yogurt, made with 1/2 cup sunflower seeds and 1/2 cup pine nuts
1 banana, mango or 1/2 papaya
3 T. fresh mint or 1 T. dried mint
1/2 " peeled ginger root
2-3 pitted dates
1 to 1 1/2 cups water

Sunflower Seed Yogurt - We Love Your Body Style

In a blender, grind:

1 cup sunflower seeds

Add:

1 cup water or 1/2 cup water and 1/2 cup Rejuvelac (2-day old, fermented soak water from wheatberries)

Blend on high until smooth and creamy like heavy cream. Pour into a glass container, cover loosely and set in a warm place until it gets thick, approximately 4-6 hours. Pour off the liquid or 'whey.' Refrigerate.

Variation: Substitute almonds, Brazil nuts, pine nuts, or 1/4 to 1/2 cup sesame seeds for the sunflower seeds.

Use this yogurt in the following ways:

Dip: Mix yogurt with chopped tomatoes, onions and celery. Add herbs, crushed garlic and sea salt or kelp. Or mix with a little grated carrot, grated beet and your favorite herbs.

Dressing: Mix yogurt with mashed avocado, chopped green onion, a little lemon juice, garlic granules and 1 t. tamari sauce. Spoon over a sprout salad.

Fruit Topping: Mix yogurt with grated apple, mashed banana, a little lemon juice and maple syrup. Mix in a little cinnamon or poppy seeds.

Tip: Seed or nut yogurts/cheeses can be used in: dips, dressings, sauces, salads, soups, shakes and smoothies. Flavor with: vanilla, almond extract, maple syrup, dates, raisins, sunflower sprouts, dried fruit, fresh fruit, ground nuts, cinnamon, nutmeg, and herbs for dips or dressings.

Seed Cheeses

Seed cheese is high in living enzymes and vitamins, especially if part or all of the water used is Rejuvelac (fermented water from wheatberries soaking). This aids in digestion. Experiment with different combinations of nuts and seeds. Cashews and macadamia nuts make a creamy cheese, alone, or blended with almonds or sunflower seeds.

> Try 1 part sunflower seeds to 1 part cashews; 1 part almonds to 1/2 part pumpkin seeds and 1/2 part macadamia nuts; 1 part almonds to 1/2 part sunflower seeds and 1/2 part walnuts; 1 part pumpkin and 1 part pecan; or 1 part sunflower seeds to 1 part pine nuts.

Generic Seed or Nut Cheese

Blend 2 cups soaked nuts and/or seeds (try 1 cup cashews, 1 cup almonds or sunflower seeds) and herbal seasonings with enough water to make a heavy cream consistency. Begin with 1 cup water. Gradually pour in up to 2 more cups or until a heavy cream texture. Place in a jar with cheesecloth or screen on top. Let set uncovered in a warm place (70-90 degrees F.). Check after 6-8 hours. If you want yogurt, pour off the "whey" and eat or refrigerate. To make cheese - turn jar upside down on a rack over a bowl and let "whey" drip out until it is of cheese consistency. This can be done in the refrigerator or at room temperature. Wrap cheese in a cheese cloth and squeeze excess "whey" off, using clean cheesecloth. Let "dry" in the refrigerator.

Ways to Use 'Cheeses'

1. To stuff Super Sushi Cones, celery, tomatoes, red pepper cups, Super Sushi Rolls, lettuce/cabbage roll-ups
2. To spread on crackers, Chapatis, Crisp Buckwheat Frisbees, dried chips
3. To spread on apple slices

Ways to Season 'Cheeses'

You can season your cheese when blending seeds and nuts with water, OR you can work in the seasonings after the cheese is completed. Your call.

1. Add garlic, onion, herbs and aminos to taste.
2. Blend with grated veggies for a dressing.
3. Add sweet spices for a sweeter 'cream' cheese.
4. Add 1/2 cup carrot pulp, 1 T. lemon juice and a little garlic.

5. Mix with minced onion, diced red pepper and grated carrot.
6. Mix with green onion, minced ginger and parsley.
7. Mash in 5 pitted dates and 1/2 t. cinnamon.
8. Add fresh, minced ginger, 1 garlic clove, minced, 1 t. dried oregano, 1/4 cup fresh basil, 1/2 t. Veg-It.

Man-in-the-Moon Green Cheese

Blend 1/2 cup chickpea (garbanzo bean) sprouts with a little water or lemon juice. Add 1/4 to 1/2 avocado and 1 t. sea salt or kelp. Mash in 1/4 cup Generic Seed or Nut Cheese. Serve over greens.

Lani's Tomatillo Salsa Rocks

3 small to medium tomatillos, cut in quarters
1/8 cup water
1/3 cup chopped, white onion
1 lime, juiced (this was not in the ingredient list on the organic salsa, but it so enlivens the salsa, I added it to this recipe)
1 T. plus 1/2 t. apple cider vinegar
1 clove garlic, peeled
1/2 jalapeño pepper, cut lengthwise and seeded (more if a hotter salsa is desired)
1/4 cup tightly-packed cilantro, leaves only
1/4 t. cumin
a few shakes of sea salt (or to taste)

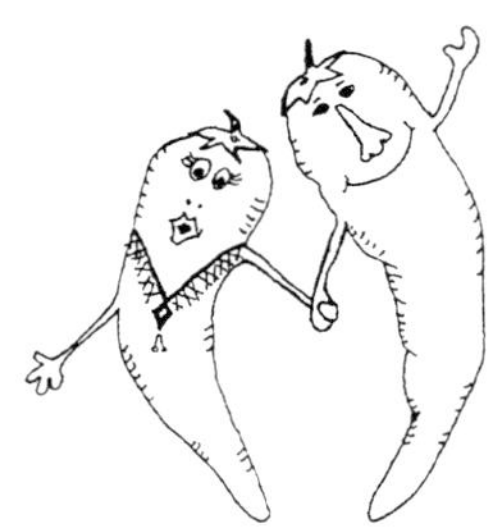

Blend all together in blender using pulses, until it is just chopped.

Add:

1/4 t. psyllium powder (to slightly thicken)

Stir and refrigerate in covered container. Makes approximately 1 cup salsa. This salsa is not too spicy or hot, and is great for spooning over green salads, sushi rolls or anything you like. You can spice up by adding more onion, cilantro or pepper. Tomatillos are slightly sweet, like green tomatoes, but with their own flavor.

Tip: If you love little Japanese-type paper lanterns, you'll love the little pod-like, paper-like calyx of the tomatillo. They added to the beauty of my Easter dinner centerpiece.

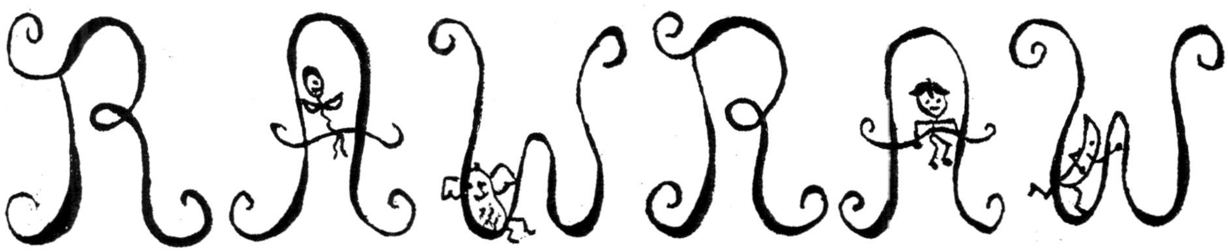

CHAPTER VII
VERSATILE VEGGIES/FABULOUS FRUITS
(SALADS, DRESSINGS, PICKLED VEGGIES, SEA VEGETABLES, SOUPS, CONDIMENTS)

Vegetable Salads

My Big Basic Salad Bowl

1. Begin by half-filling a big salad bowl with Gaia's Greens, or heaping Gaia's Greens on a dinner plate.

2. Shred some red cabbage and sprinkle a layer on top of the greens.

3. Add any vegetables you so desire. Be sure to vary the way you cut the vegetables for aesthetic reasons as well as for texture, variety and to please your palate.. For example, you can dice zucchini, make matchsticks of zucchini, slice into circles, grate zucchini or even buy a kitchen tool (about $14.00) that will cut it into long, spaghetti-like strands. This works especially well with yellow, crookneck squash and other squashes.

Vegetables: radish, green onion, red onion, green cabbage, cucumber, carrots, beets, celery, jicama, diced yam, asparagus, broccoli, cauliflower, parsley, cilantro, zucchini, tomato, sweet red or green pepper, jalapeño pepper, corn taken off the cob, fresh peas, green beans

4. Top with Sprouts: alfalfa, clover, spicy mix, lentil-mung-adzuki sprouts, sprouted quinoa or buckwheat, sprouted sunflower seeds

5. Sprinkle nuts and seeds: sunflower seeds, chopped walnuts, pecans, almonds, macadamia, cashew nuts, pine nuts (soaked or not). Crumble pieces of nori strips for minerals and flavor.

6. Avocado: A daily mainstay. A nutritious fat, good for your skin. Slice, dice, mash, but put it on your salad.

7. Complete the salad with a dressing, a pate, a sauce, a salsa, lemon juice and olive oil, a seed yogurt, thinned - whatever is uncooked and your favorite. Use your favorite fresh herbs in your salad dressings or chop and put on top of greens - thyme, basil, mint, oregano, rosemary, fresh ginger, garlic, dill. I like to add some dressing after the greens, then put a dollop of sauce or pate on top of the sprouts.

8. Other additions: Spoon a few tablespoons of Curried Lentil-Mung-Adzuki Sprout Salad on top of the greens for added protein, vitamins and live enzymes.

9. Finally, sit down, be in gratitude for the live plants, full of the energy of the sun, with enzymes, minerals and vitamins, transferring their energy to you - to nourish every cell in your body, for growth, maintenance and rebuilding. Eat slowly, remember to chew and don't eat at all if you are in a rush or upset in any way.

This salad is a complete meal. It can be eaten for lunch or dinner, but will most likely be eaten alone and will be your biggest meal. Accompany with sprouted bread, chips (dried veggie) or crackers.

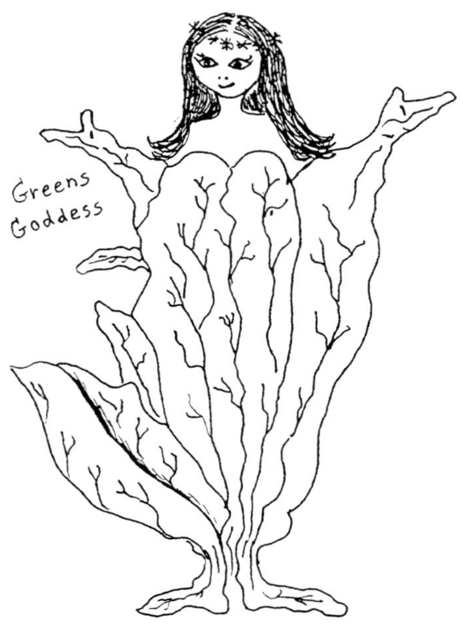

Gaia's Gift of Greens (for My Big Basic Salad Bowl)

Choose among the following greens to use as the base of your basic salad bowl:

Radicchio, escarole, tat sol, mache', frisee, lollo rosso, baby spinach, endive, chervil, mizuna, arugula, red leaf lettuce, butter lettuce, Romaine lettuce, green leafy lettuce, red Swiss chard (delicious with an olive oil and vinegar and herb dressing), sunflower lettuce, buckwheat lettuce, any other specialty lettuces, such as miner's lettuce, including parsley and cilantro. Chinese vegetables are great - bok choy, baby bok choy, mung bean sprouts, sugar snap pea pods, savoy cabbage, Napa cabbage. My preference is to never use iceberg head lettuce as a green for my salad.

Complete Protein Salad

2 cups mung bean sprouts
2 T. olive oil
1/4 cup sunflower seed meal
dash of kelp or dulse flakes

Mix together in a bowl.

Complementary Salad

2 cups alfalfa or clover sprouts
2 cups shredded Romaine lettuce
4-5 radishes, sliced
3 tomatoes, cut in 1/2 inch slices
sweet onion rings (thin) - as much as desired
1 green or red pepper, sliced in rings

Mix all together in a bowl and serve with your favorite seed sauce or dressing. An avocado dressing goes well with this salad.

Heavenly Salad

2 cups shredded red cabbage
2 cups shredded green cabbage (try savoy or Napa sometimes)
1 cup jicama, julienned
1 cup grated carrots
1 cup corn, cut off the cob

Mix all together and serve with a light dressing. In a blender place 1 avocado, sliced and the juice from 2 limes. Add about 1/4 cup water. Blend and pour over coleslaw.

Variation: Add 1/2 cup pineapple in place of carrots, reduce corn to 1/2 cup and add 1/2 cup each of julienned red pepper and yellow pepper. Make a dressing of pineapple juice and a little tahini. Or blend 1/2 cup walnut or flax oil, 1 T. apple cider vinegar, juice of one lemon and dill seed, to taste. . Garnish with walnuts or pecans, mint and parsley.

Tip: If someone in the family doesn't like certain vegetables, they can be minced very fine and added to the salad dressing. They won't even notice.

Rooty Salad

1 cup grated carrots
1/2 cup grated parsnips
2 Jerusalem artichokes (sun chokes), peeled or well-scrubbed and sliced thin
1/4 cup grated beet
4 red radishes, sliced thin

Toss all together and serve on bed of greens with avocado and lime juice dressing.

Variation: Grate zucchini or yellow crookneck squash, spaghetti squash or yams

Stuffed Tomatoes, Red Bell Peppers, Avocado or Zucchini Boats All Hollowed and Ready to Fill

Fill with Curried, Lentil-Mung-Adzuki Sprout Salad.
Fill with Hearty Party Dip.
Fill with Sunrise Sauce.
Fill with Sprouted Lentil Patties.
Fill with YOUR own mixture of sprouted lentils and mung beans mixed with chopped onion, celery, olive oil, tamari sauce, cider vinegar, kelp, cayenne, grated carrots.
Fill with Mock Tuna salad.
Fill with diced avocado, tomatoes, cilantro, onions.
Fill with diced celery, tomatoes, chopped walnuts, salad dressing of your choice.
Fill with clover or alfalfa sprouts, kelp and a little lime juice.
Fill with diced celery and a little seed cheese.
Fill with guacamole and top with torn lettuce leaves.

Salad Burrito

Grind 1/2 cup sunflower seed sprouts and 1/2 cup soaked, raw almonds. Mix with an olive oil and lemon juice dressing, finely chopped tomatoes, drained, and diced, sweet onion. Form a stiff roll and place on an open Romaine or red lettuce leaf. Sprinkle with alfalfa or clover sprouts and roll up like a burrito.

Broccoli-in-Bed

2 cups broccoli florets, finely chopped

Place in a bowl. In a measuring cup, make a marinade:

2 T. olive oil

2 t. tamari sauce

1 lime or 1/2 lemon, juiced

Mix marinade and pour over broccoli, stirring well. Cover and refrigerate for at least 6 hours to tenderize the broccoli. When ready to serve, pour off the marinade.

Serve as a side dish with Hearty Party Dip or Sunrise Sauce spooned over it, or spoon broccoli on top of your big salad with the sauce mixed into it.

Variation: To the chopped broccoli add 1/2 cup raisins, thinly sliced red onion rings, chopped red pepper, green onion, sliced and 1/4 cup packed cilantro, chopped. Toss together with Sunrise Sauce or Orange Dressing. Chill, then sprinkle on some sunflower seeds just before serving.

Karli's Peace Salad

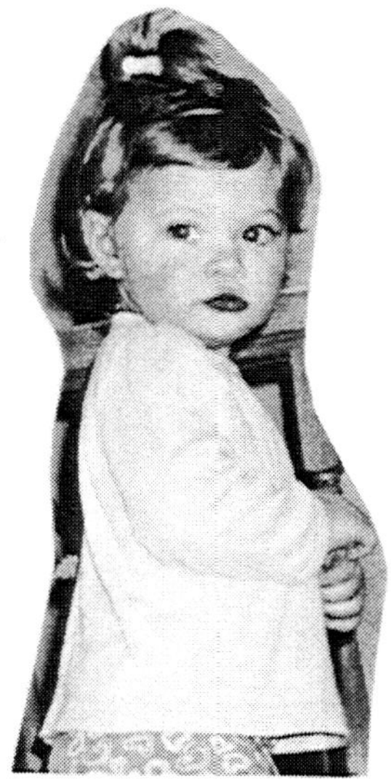

red cabbage, grated
carrots, grated
red leaf lettuce
cucumber circles
tomato slices
sunflower seed sprouts

Prepare vegetables. On a salad plate, create salad as follows:

Place a handful of torn lettuce and chard. Form an 'X' across the salad using a thin line of grated carrots going in one direction and a line of grated, red cabbage in the other direction, completing the 'X'. Place a thin tomato slice or wedge on top of the center of the 'X'. Place 4 cucumber slices at the edge of the salad plate, two to the left of the 'X' and two to the right. Sprinkle a few sunflower seeds or sunflower seed sprouts on top of the salad. Drizzle over the salad your child's favorite salad dressing.

This salad has a little history. I had gone down to Mt. Shasta to help a friend prepare food for a formal dinner party. She was having a peace dialog. Fourteen or fifteen ministers, pastors, priests, reverends and monks had been invited to speak their views about peace--peace in the world, their community and how they practiced peace in their own lives. Members of the community were invited to come after dinner to listen to the peace dialog and interact after each religious leader had spoken their views.

There were several of us there preparing a grand dinner. The monks had come over from India, with an interpreter. Two tables were set up beautifully for the dinner. The people at one table were being served vegetarian food, while the monks and several people at their table were being served a meat dinner (at their request). All were being served the same dinner salad, which I volunteered to prepare. We wanted something simple and colorful, as well as tasty. My friend mentioned that the monks were not used to salad or fresh, uncooked salad ingredients. I bought two kinds of greens (red leaf lettuce, and green leaf lettuce). I sliced cucumbers, grated red cabbage and carrots. I sliced Roma tomatoes, then began to prepare each small salad plate. We formed an 'X' on top of the greens with the grated carrots and cabbage, placed the tomato slice on top and cucumber slices to the sides. Then an Italian dressing was drizzled over all. The salad looked appetizing and fortunately, most of the monks ate their salad.

A day after the dinner, I drove north to Portland to visit my daughter and her family, 19-month old Karli and 9 year old Jake. For two dinner meals, I prepared salads for everyone, using the leftover ingredients. Karli, who had not been offered green salads in her life, was sitting on my lap. She had already been fed. However, she took one look at everyone's salad and watched us eating them. Suddenly, she plunged her little fingers into my salad, first chewing on a cucumber slice, then discovering the grated carrot, the grated cabbage, sunflower seeds and the mixed greens. Placing fingers full of salad ingredients into her mouth, she enjoyed over half of my salad.

This just illustrates how much toddlers can enjoy raw, living food. Most toddlers are used to fresh, mashed or sliced fruit, but not as many eat raw veggies, other than carrot slices. If they have teeth, they can attempt to chew some salad ingredients. Be sure to offer a variety to them and let them pick and choose according to their tastes. Sometimes it is the texture that they are not fond of, but add a dressing they enjoy and they'll be dipping those carrot, zucchini, or cucumbers slices into the dip or dressing and benefiting from the living food. Sometimes it is so easy to open a jar of baby food or prepare an easy noodle or rice dish. However, kids need living food as much as adults for a healthy digestive system and flora. Have it available for them whenever they are served to the adults.

Triple Grated Salad

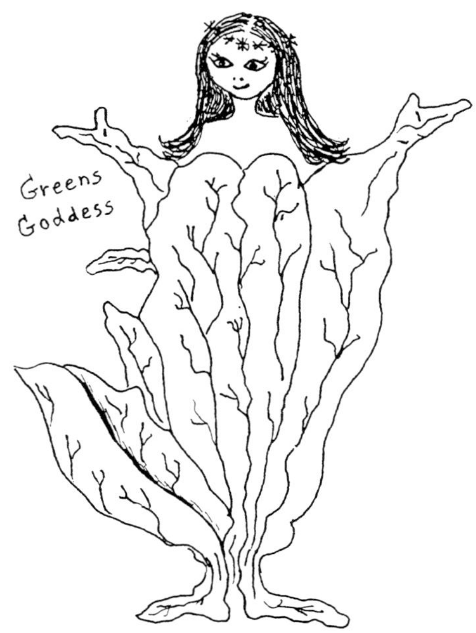

Make separate mounds on a plate of greens with the following:

2 grated carrots
2 grated beets
1 cup grated Napa or savoy cabbage
1/2 cup finely chopped parsley

Drizzle a tahini dressing over all.

Quinoa Tabouleh

1/2 cup sprouted quinoa
3/4 cup chopped tomatoes (chop and allow to drain in a strainer before adding to salad)
1 T. tamari sauce
1/4 cup lemon juice (the juice from 1 medium lemon)
1 T. chopped, fresh mint, packed
1/4 cup finely chopped white onion (or 1-2 green onions, sliced thin)
1/4 cup heaped with diced cucumber
3/4 cup chopped parsley (loosely packed)
1 t. minced jalapeño pepper
1 t. minced fresh ginger, peeled
1/4 cup olive oil (optional-add anywhere from 2 T. to 1/2 cup olive oil)

Place all ingredients in a bowl. Stir well after each addition. May be a little juicy. Can drain off extra juice before serving.

Refrigerate, covered, at least 2 hours before serving to allow flavors to blend. Overnight refrigeration is best.

Jicama Salad

Julienne or matchstick the following: 1 small carrot, 1 small zucchini with skin on (not the center seeds), 1 small red bell pepper and 1 small yellow bell pepper, seeded, 1 small jicama, peeled. Dice one-fourth of a seeded jalapeño. Place all in a bowl.

In a small bowl, mix together: 2-3 T. olive oil and 1/2 lime, juiced, sea salt to taste. Pour over veggies and toss several times to mix.

Curried Lentil-Mung-Adzuki Sprout Salad

This tasty salad is easy to make (sprouting takes only 2-3 days) and is great alone as a salad or added as a topping to any green salad. It can be plain or add your favorite lemon juice/olive oil dressing or miso dressing.

1/4 cup raw sunflower seeds - sprouted 1-2 days
About 2 cups total of lentil sprouts, adzuki sprouts and mung sprouts
1/4 t. sea salt
1/2 t. curry powder
2 celery stalks, finely diced
1/2 to 1 t. minced jalapeño pepper
1-3 green onions, sliced thin

Mix all of the above into a salad bowl.

In a blender place 1 chopped garlic clove, 2-3 T. olive oil, 2 T. lemon juice. Blend until smooth and pour over salad. Stir well, cover and refrigerate until ready to use. Makes a good filling when mixed with alfalfa or clover sprouts and put into hollowed-out avocado halves, tomatoes or green or red bell peppers, cutting the pepper in half lengthwise for two boats or cutting it in half crosswise for a small cup shape.

Juicy, Rainbow Salad

In one big bowl, place the following:

red leaf lettuce, broken into bite size pieces
big handful of organic, spring mix (all kinds of greens)
big handful clover sprouts (well-rinsed)
1 celery stalk, diced

In food processor, using grater attachment, grate:

1 small zucchini
1 small, yellow, crookneck squash
1 carrot
a wedge or two of red cabbage

Add the grated mixture to salad and mix with hands until blended. (Sometimes I leave on top)

Dressings: Over one-half the salad, spoon out some of Lani's Tomatillo Salsa Rocks. Over the other half, pour some Orange Avocado Dressing for Greens. This is a very delicious, juicy, nutritious salad.

Wild & Wonderful Green, Green Salad

miner's lettuce, several handfuls, washed, dried and cut into thirds (use Romaine or red leaf as substitute)
spring greens or washed, baby spinach
handful of cilantro, cut into thirds (or remove stems, your choice)
diced celery, 1 or two stalks
diced cucumber - 1/3 cucumber
diced jicama
Roma tomato, cut into small slices
a few chopped cashew nuts

Dressing: Over one half the salad, spoon Lani's Tomatillo Salsa Rocks. Over the other half, spoon or dollop either Mi Miso Dressing, or a black olive dressing. Delicious!!

Super Sprout Salad

In any amounts, mix chopped buckwheat lettuce, sunflower greens, sunflower seed sprouts, alfalfa or clover sprouts, a handful of mixed sprouts (garbanzo, lentil, adzuki, mung, soy) chopped green onion, grated carrot, diced celery, diced cucumber, chopped avocado and mushrooms. Toss with your favorite dressing or a lemon juice and oil dressing and garnish with tomato wedges. Sprinkle kelp and cayenne over all.

Colorful Veggie Kebobs

Thread zucchini chunks, cherry tomatoes, avocado cubes, mushrooms, cucumber chunks, black olives, rutabaga slices, Jerusalem artichoke chunks, green olives, etc., onto bamboo skewers. Have your favorite dressing to drizzle over. Place on bed of greens.

Super Duper Sprout Salad

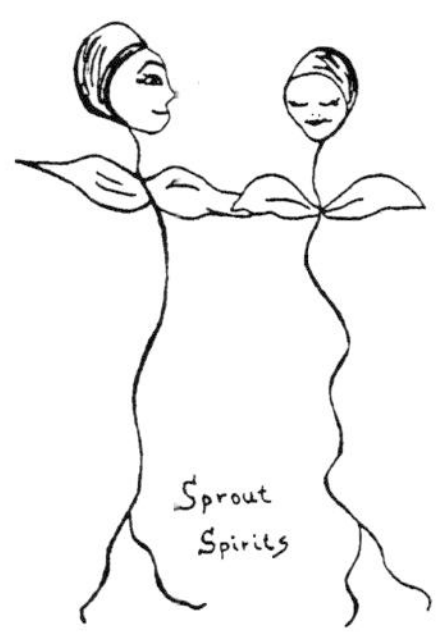

alfalfa sprouts
radish sprouts
sunflower seed sprouts
grated carrot
grated beet
fresh lemon juice
powdered kelp
avocado

In a salad bowl place a small handful of alfalfa sprouts. Sprinkle a few radish sprouts around the alfalfa sprouts. On top of the sprouts, place about 1 T. sunflower seed sprouts. Top with the desired amount of grated carrot and beet. Juice a lemon and drizzle a little lemon over the salad. Sprinkle with powdered kelp and drizzle Pineapple-Cream Dressing over all. Garnish with diced avocado or avocado slices.

Tip: Use parsley often as it is high in vitamin C. It keeps well in a jar in the refrigerator or can be dried. Tie a bunch and hang upside down or place sprigs on dehydrator sheet and dry just until no moisture is left.

Soup Can Cylinders

Choose any number below to layer your cylinder, usually 1/2" to 1" layers. Open a clean, empty soup can at both ends. Oil inside of can and place upright on cutting board. Carefully and gently, pack each layer into the soup can. When ready to serve, use a spatula under soup can to move to salad plate. Using a table knife, carefully loosen the mixture along the edges, if necessary, and lift can off the mixture. You should see a lovely layered salad. Drizzle your favorite dressing over and serve surrounded with greens and grated veggies.

#1. Layer with a) diced red tomatoes/diced onion; b) chopped zucchini/basil, Bragg's aminos; and c) your favorite guacamole. Repeat layers until tower is as tall as you want. Move to plate and surround with clover sprouts and fresh salsa. Have dehydrated zucchini chips nearby.

#2. Layer with these combinations: a) diced yellow tomato with sliced green onion, cilantro and 1 t. each lemon juice and olive oil; b) diced red tomato with chives, basil and 1 t. each lemon juice and olive oil; c) cubed avocado with lime juice drizzled over. When there are several packed layers of each, move can to plate. Carefully remove can and serve with sprouts all around.

#3. Your favorite pate or hummus, alternated with packed, chopped alfalfa sprouts drizzled with lemon juice and Bragg's aminos. Serve on plate with diced tomatoes and cucumbers with lime wedges and cilantro leaves.

Nests

Grate some carrots, cabbage. Add diced celery. Mix in a bowl with a little sesame or olive oil and 1 t. apple cider vinegar. In individual bowls, spoon this mixture in and press against sides of bowls to form nests. Fill with seed sauce or yogurt. Top with chopped buckwheat lettuce, sunflower greens or Captain Buckwheat Crunch.

Christmas Salad

1 cup red cabbage, grated
1 beet, grated
1/2 to 3/4 cup baby peas (frozen is okay)
2 T. jalapeno pepper, seeded
1/2 lime, juiced
1/4 t. onion powder or granules
1/4 t. garlic powder or granules

Toss all together and refrigerate.

Vegetable Salad Dressings

Papaya Dressing

In a blender, blend until smooth:

1/2 of a ripe papaya
1/2 lime, juiced
1/2 t. dry mustard
dash sea salt
2 T. water

Refrigerate until needed.

Oil and Lemon or Vinegar Herb Dressing

1/3 cup olive oil
1/2 lemon, juiced OR 1-3 T. apple cider vinegar
your choice of fresh basil, or dried herbs
1 garlic clove, minced

Blend all together in blender. Refrigerate.

Orange Avocado Dressing for Greens

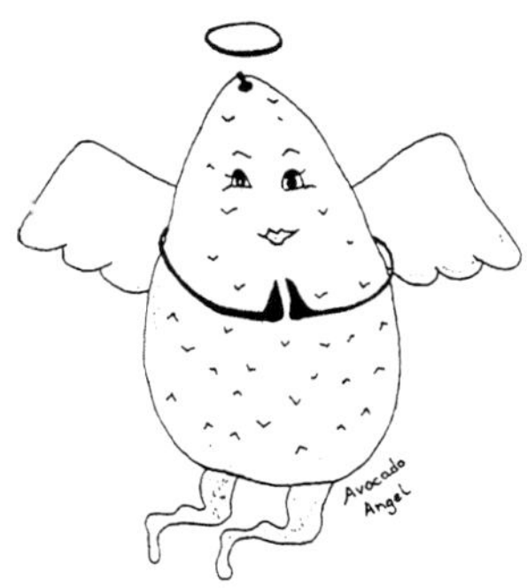

1 avocado
1 orange, juiced
1/2 to 1 t. tamari sauce or Nama Shoyu

Blend in a blender until smooth. Use immediately.

Avocado and Carrot Juice Dressing

Blend one avocado with some carrot juice for a delicious green salad dressing. May add herbs as desired.

Tip: When selecting salad ingredients, consider: texture combinations (some soft, some crunchy), variety in color and taste, protein quality, produce in season, whether a main dish or side salad, and type of dressing to be used.

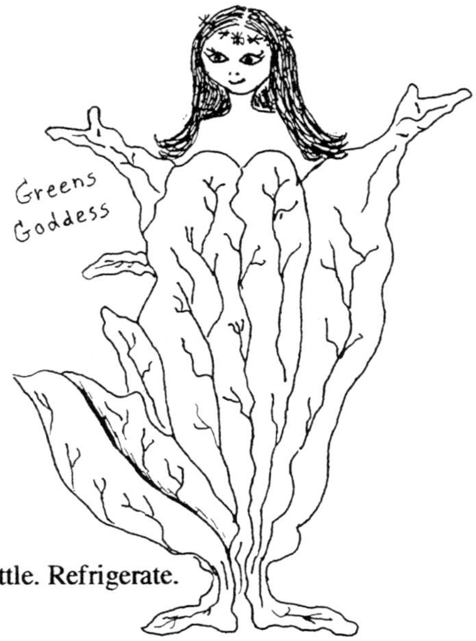

Mi Miso Dressing

1 cup water
1/4" slice ginger root, peeled and minced
5 T. tahini
2-3 T. white miso
1/2 to 1 lemon, juiced
1-2 T. sweet onion

Blend all in a blender until smooth. Pour into a plastic ketchup bottle. Refrigerate.

Ashland Food Cooperative Miso Dressing

In a blender, blend the following ingredients until smooth:

1 cup plus 2 T. white miso, 1/2 cup plus 2 T. shoyu sauce, 1/2 cup plus 2 T. apple cider vinegar, 1/2 cup plus 2 T. water, 2 cups plus 3 T. safflower oil, 3/4 cup plus 1 T. chopped, yellow onion (Freely given by the Food Cooperative-I divided ingredients by 3 to yield less for home use)

Green Goddess Dressing

Blend all ingredients in a blender until smooth.

1-2 avocados
1-2 garlic cloves
1-2 lemons, juiced
1/4 to 1/2 cup chopped parsley
2 green onions, sliced
1/2 t. tamari sauce or to taste

Add water as needed to make creamy.

Variation: In place of lemon juice, garlic and onions, substitute lime juice and minced sweet onion. Keep refrigerated in covered container.

Avocado Sweet & Spicy Dressing

In a blender, blend:

1/2 avocado
3 T. lemon juice
1 T. raisins
pinch of cayenne pepper
water to blend smoothly

French Dressing

In a blender, blend:

1 cup olive oil
1/3 cup apple cider vinegar
1 T. maple syrup
1/2 t. garlic powder or granules
1/4 t. sea salt
1/4 t. paprika
1/8 t. dry mustard powder
dash of cayenne pepper
1 small tomato, chopped

Black Olive Dressing Challenge

These are the ingredients on a bottle of fresh, unpasteurized olive dressing I bought at a local farmer's market. Try to duplicate with substitutions and omissions this tasty dressing:

Ingredients: soybean oil, rice vinegar, black olives, soy protein, fresh garlic, purified water, salt, pepper

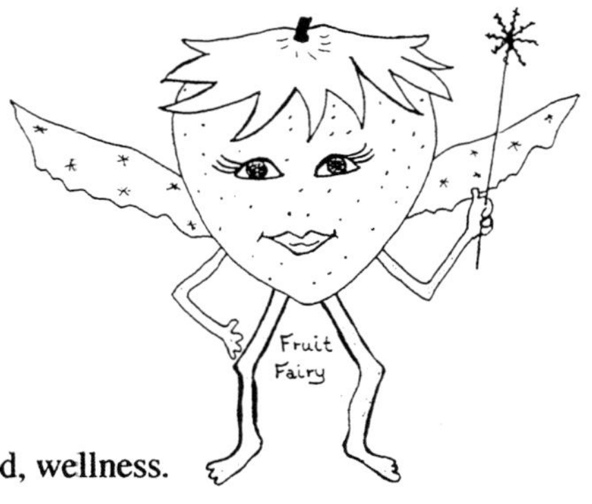

Fruit Salads

Mandalas

Mandalas are symbols of oneness, wholeness, and when applied to food, wellness.

Preparing your greens, vegetables or fruits onto a platter in a mandala-like pattern, adds a special aesthetic appeal to your guests and your artistic spirit. It allows for choice, as the guests can choose the variety offered to them and form their own small mandala on a greens-lined plate.

Begin with a large platter. In the center place a small bowl containing the dressing, sauce or puree for the fruits or veggies. Form a 'cross' to make four quadrants or make three lines to make 6 even divisions.

For a vegetable platter, try finely grated beets, carrots and red cabbage to make the line divisions. Fill in the six areas with a variety of diced, wedged, grated, julienned, veggies for a colorful mandala, keeping each section separate.

Sample: 1. torn, red Swiss chard 2. wedge-cut yellow squash 3. cucumber sticks 4. diced jicama 5. miner's lettuce, butter lettuce or sprouts 6. tomato wedges

For a fruit platter, try sliced apples, dried cherries and tangerine boats to make the divisions. Fill in the six areas with a variety of soaked, dried fruit and fresh fruit. There are dozens of combinations possible:

Sample: 1. soaked, dried plums 2. kiwi slices 3. fresh, whole strawberries 4. fresh figs, cut in half 5. sliced bananas, drizzled with lime juice 6. green or red grapes

Variation: Arrange fruit or veggies (keep greens on individual plates) in concentric circles for a pretty mandala, leaving out the pie-shaped divisions. Keep the larger veggies (slices or wedges on the outer circles and the smaller, grated or matchstick fruits or veggies toward the center. Place the bowl of dressing or sauce in the center.

In April, after being on a live food eating plan for nearly four months, I went to a five day healing prayer retreat, where only vegetarian food was served. There were 16 people eating together, three meals a day plus snacks. I brought some of my own food (nuts, Marbles, Sunrise Sauce, some fruit); however, I relied on the two cooks to prepare my meals. I asked them to prepare salads and fruits for me. These two, wonderful people gave me more than that. Each meal was a plate of color, texture, and art--all done mandala-style. Many of the other participants in the retreat looked enviously at my platter. The mandalas included raisins, dried cranberries, citrus boats, sliced pears, apples or bananas, whole, raw almonds. The veggie mandalas were arranged beautifully using sliced avocadoes, mixed, raw nuts, grated carrots, celery slices, cucumber circles, mixed greens, and tomato slices. It was a pleasure and joy to be eating these in such a peaceful, beautiful environment.

Spices to Dress up a Fruit Salad

cinnamon, nutmeg, crushed anise, mace, cardamom, allspice

Start with just a dash and add more to taste. Try only one at a time to see how it enhances the natural flavor of the fruit.

Confetti Salad

This colorful salad is made in any amount in the following proportions:

3 parts orange or tangelo slices, cut into thirds
2 parts fresh strawberries, sliced
1 part kiwis, peeled and sliced into rounds.

Mix all together in a bowl with 2 T. lime juice. Refrigerate covered, then stir again just before serving.

Variation: Add 1/2 banana, sliced and a sprinkle of cinnamon.

Colorful Fruit Kebobs

Thread orange wedges, banana chunks (brushed with lime juice to prevent discoloring), apple wedges (brushed with lime juice), apricot halves, pear slices, pineapple chunks, green or red grapes, cantaloupe or watermelon chunks, nectarine slices, etc. onto bamboo skewers. Serve on a plate with shredded greens. About 2 skewers per person makes a nice luncheon. Drizzle with your favorite fruit dressing.

Super Vitamin-Packed Fruit Breakfast

In a large bowl, mix:

2-3 peeled bananas, sliced
2 apples, sliced
1-2 oranges, sliced

Spoon into individual salad bowls. Pour Pineapple Orange Dressing over all.

Variation: Substitute Sweet Yogurt Dressing for Pineapple Orange Dressing.

Aloha Salad

Blend 1 cup chunky, sliced pineapple to desired consistency.

Pour over:

1 large handful alfalfa or clover sprouts
1/4 cup sunflower seed meal (about 3 T. sunflower seeds, ground to a fine powder)

Waldorf Salad

apples, chopped
walnuts
green or purple grapes
golden currants or raisins
celery, diced
sunflower seeds, sprouted

Mix in a large bowl in your favorite proportions. Then make this dressing and spoon over or mix in. Crushed, fresh pineapple mixed in with 1 cup nut or seed yogurt. Stir well. Sprinkle salad with allspice.

Dressy Pineapple Rings

Slice a fresh pineapple into rings, with the core and outer skin removed. Place each ring on a salad plate with greens. Spoon into the center of each ring a dollop of the following mixture:

1 peeled orange, cubed
1 avocado, cubed
1/4 cup shredded, unsweetened coconut
1 T. honey
dash of cinnamon

Pineapple Boat

Cut a fresh pineapple in half lengthwise through the crown. Remove a lot of the fruit, leaving skin intact. Core and dice the fruit. In a bowl, toss the pineapple with 2 cups fresh strawberries, 1 cup sliced celery, 1/2 cup chopped walnuts, 1/2 cup green grapes, 1/4 cup sunflower seeds or sunflower seed sprouts.

Spoon mixture back into the pineapple boats and serve with your favorite fruit sauce or dressing

Party Fruit Salad

Alternate peeled slices of cantaloupe, honeydew melon and avocado on a bed of lettuce leaves. Drizzle with Orange-Cashew Cream. Optional: Sprinkle with fresh raspberries and shredded coconut.

Fruit Salad Dressings and Sauces

Delicious Dried Fruit Purees

Try these fruit purees to use as sauces or dressings over fruit salads:

Use dried plums, cherries, raisins, apricots or any combination.

Basic Recipe: In a food processor, using 'S' blade, process until smooth:

1 cup dried, pitted fruit

1 cup water

When smooth, add a little vanilla, cinnamon or orange zest for flavor. Pour over Muesli or fresh fruit for additional nutrition and flavor.

Ambrosia Dressing

In a blender, blend well:

fruit of 1/2 papaya

1/2 lime, juiced

pinch sea salt

1 t. honey

Drizzle over fruit kebobs or fruit salad.

Pineapple-Cream Dressing

Blend 3/4 to 1 cup fresh pineapple chunks with 3-4 T. cashews until creamy.

Pineapple Orange Dressing

In a blender, blend:

1 1/2 cups fresh pineapple chunks

1/2 cup fresh orange juice

Pour sauce over salads.

Garnish with your choice of the following:

finely chopped almonds, sunflower seed sprouts, chopped dates

Tahini Fruit Dressing

Blend well in a blender:

1 cup tahini
2 oranges, juiced
2 dates, pitted
1/2 t. Five Spice Powder

Add only enough water to keep the dressing smooth and creamy.

Sweet Tahini Sauce

In a blender, blend 1 ripe banana, 1/4 cup raw tahini and a little fruit juice to make a thick sauce. (Apple juice is great.) Pour sauce over a bowl of sliced bananas or other fruit. Garnish with soaked golden raisins or apples and a dash of cinnamon.

Date Orange Sauce (for fruit salads)

In a blender, pour 1 cup warm water and 2 cups pitted, chopped dates. Soak until dates are soft. Add 1 cup orange juice and blend together.

Two Sweet Yogurt Dressings

1. Stir together gently 1 cup Cinn-fully Delicious Yogurt, 1 T. Almond-Cinnamon Mixture, 1/4 cup chopped, pitted dates and 2 T. fresh orange juice.

2. Stir together gently 1 cup Cinn-fully Delicious Yogurt with 1 t. vanilla, 1 T. honey, 1 T. maple syrup and 2 T. lime or lemon juice. Chill.

Orange-Cashew Cream

Blend 1 cup each orange juice and washed cashew nuts until smooth. Add a dash of nutmeg, mace or 5 Spice Powder to enhance the flavor.

Pickled Veggies

Pickled Onions

2 red onions, thinly sliced
1/4 c. lemon juice

Refrigerate in glass jar, and shake occasionally.

Marinated Mushrooms

1 lb. sliced mushrooms (I like shitake)
1 garlic clove, minced
2 T. olive oil
1/4 cup lemon juice
1 t. oregano
1/4 cup chopped, fresh parsley
Bragg's aminos, to taste (sparingly)

Mix all in a bowl and let sit for at least an hour.

Marinated Chickpeas

Marinate sprouted chickpeas in olive oil, lemon juice, parsley, minced garlic clove, dash of nutmeg, salt and cayenne pepper. Sprinkle over salad or eat as a side dish.

Marinated Cucumbers

2 cucumbers, sliced thin (don't peel, if organic)
1/2 red onion, sliced thin
2 T. lemon juice
2 T. fresh parsley, finely chopped
dash of tumeric powder
dash of cayenne pepper
1 t. minced garlic
Bragg's aminos, to taste

Mix all in a bowl and let sit an hour before serving.

Raw Slaw

Mix finely chopped cabbage with thin-sliced radishes, fresh dill, apple cider vinegar and olive oil. Marinate for a couple of hours. Then add a little honey or apple juice to sweeten and chill.

Sea Vegetables

Seaweeds, also called sea vegetables, grow naturally in the ocean along the coasts of continents. They are a rich source of vitamins and enzymes as well as minerals. Some of the concentrated vitamins and minerals, to name a few, are calcium, magnesium, vitamins A, B, D, E and K. Sea vegetables are healing to the joints, mucous membranes and skin. Try to buy organic since their source is usually in the clear, unpolluted waters of Northern Canada, Norway or Iceland.

When harvested fresh, sea vegetables do not need to be reconstituted. However, most are purchased dried and must be soaked for approximately 15 minutes, then rinsed and drained. This is to remove some of the salt and any other residue, such as bits of shells, or sea life. Some popular varieties that can be eaten raw are as follows:

Nori - usually formed into sheets for nori rolls or sushi. Can be crumbled onto salads. Does not require soaking if purchased in sheets. Purchase untoasted for a truly raw food.

Sea Palm - for salads

Hijiki - for salads

Wakame - for salads

Dulse - for snacks, salads, powdered or granulated to sprinkle over anything; dehydrated to eat in salads

Hip Hip Hijiki Salad

3/4 cup hijiki, dried (soak for 15 min., rinse in water and drain)
1 carrot, finely grated
1 cup finely shredded green cabbage
2/3 cup lentil sprouts
2 T. lemon juice
1 T. apple cider vinegar
3 green onions, sliced thinly (tops included)
1 T. aminos
1 T. sunflower seeds (regular or sprouted)
1 t. tamari sauce
1 t. sesame seeds

Place all ingredients in a bowl except for the sesame seeds. Chill. Garnish with sesame seeds and parsley and serve.

Super Sushi Rolls

For filling: Use Hearty Party Dip, Oregon Hummus or any crumbled patty mixed with my miso dressing for a filling. Spread onto a sheet of nori. If using Yummy Yammy Patties, do the following: In a bowl, crumble about 2 patties. Add chopped celery, 1 radish diced, a few sunflower seeds, a few T. of diced red onion. Add 1-2 T. flax or olive oil. Mix by hand until consistency of a spread. Spread over half a nori sheet which is on a bamboo mat or a plate.

Make match sticks or thin slices of the following to place over filling, parallel to end of nori sheet closest to you (the short side): carrots, sweet red pepper, slices of avocado, green onion (including tops).

Have alfalfa or clover sprouts washed and dried ready.

Procedure:

1. Lay your untoasted nori sheet on a plate or bamboo mat, shortest end closest to you.
2. Spread the filling on half of the nori sheet closest to you.
3. Lay out sticks of veggies parallel to the end of nori sheet, just about 2" in from end, three or four in a line. Example: 1 avocado slice, 1 red pepper stick, 1 green onion in lengthwise slivers, 1 carrot stick, then move on down and repeat until you get to end of sheet.
4. Squirt miso dressing over all.
5. Spread alfalfa or clover sprouts over far half of nori sheet.
6. Begin by rolling up tightly, rolling over the veggie sticks on past the rest of the filling and over the sprouts. Seal with water along the far end of the nori sheet. It should stick to itself and seal.

Serve within an hour before nori gets soggy and absorbs the moisture of the filling. Wrap in plastic wrap and take with you for lunch at work or a picnic. Keep in a cooler. Or take a serrated knife and cut into slightly diagonal slices – 2-4 per roll and place upright on plate of greens.

Super Sushi Cones

Cut nori sheets in triangles and roll like a cone. Fill with seed sauce or yogurt, sprouts, avocado and carrot/red pepper sticks

Tip: Using plastic zip-lock bags, grate carrots and red cabbage separately and place in the bags. You will have enough for salads for several days and won't have to get out the grater each time you want a salad. You can do the same with cucumbers, radishes, green onions, zucchini, lettuces, red peppers. Wash the veggies, then store in a tight container in the refrigerator. When needed they are easily available for quick preparation.

Super Sushi, Cabbage, or Lettuce Rolls

Fillings for lettuce, cabbage or sushi rolls
your favorite seed cheese (i.e., Hearty Party Dip, Sprouted Sunflower Seed Cheese)
tomato slices
avocado
cilantro sprigs
clover sprouts, alfalfa sprouts
tomatoes, diced
baby spinach leaves
your favorite dressing

Spread lettuce, cabbage leaf or nori sheet with dip or seed cheese. Layer with avocado slices, tomatoes and sprouts. Press spinach leaves on top and roll tightly. Moisten end of nori sheet to seal, or seal lettuce or cabbage rolls with toothpick.

Carrot Hijiki Salad

1/2 small yam, grated
2 carrots, grated
1 small red or yellow pepper, cut in strips
a handful of clover sprouts
1/4 cup pine nuts, soaked
1/4 cup hijiki, soaked for at least 10 minutes; then rinse and discard soak water

Place in a bowl and mix with a spoon. Line a clean salad bowl with greens. Spoon in the salad. Pour an avocado dressing over the salad, or use tamari sauce with lemon juice and honey.

'Tuna'-4-2

In food processor, using 'S' blade, process the following:

1/2 cup raw, soaked almonds, blanched (pour water that has boiled over almonds for a minute)
1-2 t. kelp powder
1/2 cup sunflower seeds (sprouted or regular raw)
1/2 cup celery, chopped

Then add the following:

1/4 cup chopped white onion
1/4 cup parsley
1/4 cup lemon juice
1 t. VegeSal or any multi-herb seasoning
1/2 cup mung bean sprouts, rinsed

Process by pulsing food processor several times to chop parsley, mung bean sprouts and onion. Transfer to a salad bowl.

In a small bowl, place 1/2 scant cup sprouted chickpeas.
Use a masher or bottom of glass to mash the chickpeas, just enough to break the beans up. Add to salad bowl.

Cut a red bell pepper in half lengthwise and scoop out seeds. Cut each half in half again to form 4 cups. Spoon the 'tuna' mixture into the cups. Garnish with parsley, a few sunflower seeds and paprika.

This is great for stuffing a red bell pepper, or spooning on a lettuce leaf and rolling up to eat as a 'sandwich.' Can be used in hollowed-out zucchini for zucchini boats. Spread some on a Crisp Buckwheat Frisbee.

Tip: Use chopsticks to eat salads and other dishes. This will lengthen the time it takes to eat your meal, force you to eat one bite at a time and remind you to chew each bite slowly and thoroughly. Focus on all the wonderful, live ingredients in the salad. Don't watch television while eating. Make your meal an experience in taste, color, flavors and in gratitude for the wonderful fruits and vegetables available to us.

Soups

Generic Soup

Place the following ingredients in a blender and blend:
Base: 1-2 juicy vegetables: cucumber, celery, red or yellow pepper, tomato
Sweetener: 1 apple or 1/2 to 1 cup carrot juice
Greens: Add 2-4 cups of greens (sprouts, spinach, lettuces, parsley, chard, buckwheat lettuce, etc.).
Liquid: Add some water as needed.
Fat: To make creamy, add an avocado, nut butter, ground nuts, or olive oil.
Herbs: Season with your favorite herbs - tamari sauce, garlic, diced onions, aminos, dried herbs

Can add chunky veggies after soup is blended, i.e. zucchini or yellow squash, grated carrots or other veggies for variety in texture.

Miso 'Soup'

In a small bowl, put 1 t. fermented white or red miso. Pour water, (heated to no greater than 100 degrees) over the miso and stir well. Add raw peas, grated carrot and thinly sliced green onion. Eat with a spoon for a hearty, warm 'soup'.

Variation: Omit the veggies and pour water in a cup with 1 t. miso. Stir and drink as a warm tea.

Condiments

Un-Salt but Salty

Slice a bunch of organic celery into thin slices and dehydrate until dry. Put in blender and powder. Makes a great salt substitute and assimilates well.

Ketchup

In blender, blend well:
1 1/2 cups sun-dried tomatoes, soaked
1/2 cup diced, fresh tomatoes
1 T. apple cider vinegar
1 T. raisins or maple syrup
1/4 cup water
Veg-It or All Purpose Seasoning to taste

Golden Mayo

In blender, blend well:
3 T. lemon juice
1/2 cup sunflower seed yogurt
2 T. apple cider vinegar
1 garlic clove
1/2 t. aminos or tamari sauce
1/2 t. tumeric powder
1/2 t. paprika
dash cayenne

Vanilla Extract

Place 2 vanilla beans in 1 quart of inexpensive brandy. Set aside for 1-2 months. Leave beans in and it will continue to improve as you use it. (Can be done with water, but tastes better with brandy)

Powdered Veggies

Powder in your blender any dehydrated veggies. This makes a great warm broth seasoning. Seaweed is great for flavoring broth, too.

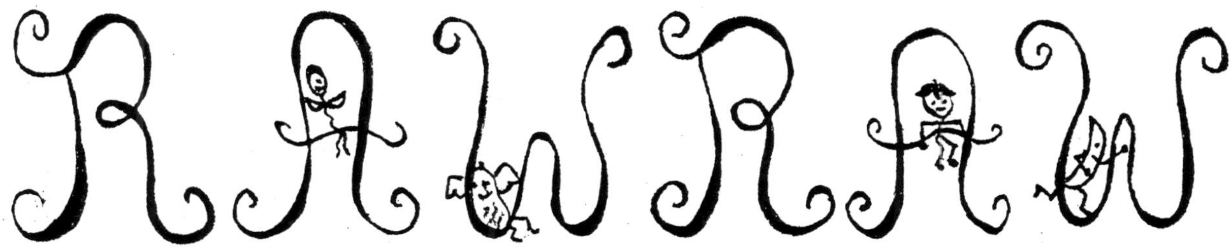

CHAPTER VIII
IT'S THE MAIN THING
PATTIES, LOAVES, MAIN DISHES

Patties

Veggie-Nut Patties

In food processor, using the 'S' blade process:

1/2 cup walnuts
a small handful of pecans

Add:

2 medium carrots - cut in quarters
1/4 cup finely grated green cabbage
2 T. grated cucumber or zucchini
1 t. raisins
2 green onions
1 t. olive oil
1/2 t. poultry seasoning
1 t. nutritional yeast

Process until well mixed. If too wet, add a little ground flax seed or dehydrated parsley or onion. Form patties, then sprinkle paprika over each. Makes 4 small patties.

Serve on a bed of lettuce. Top with a few clover or alfalfa sprouts. Place wedges or slices of tomato beside the patties. Tastes good with a dollop of Sunrise Sauce or Party Pate'.

Variation: After processing, add diced radish and celery to mixture.

Variation: For a fish patty, crumble a 2" x 4" strip of nori into mixture prior to forming patties, or 1-2 t. powdered kelp.

Yummy Yammy Patties

Using food processor with grater attachment, process:
peeled yam until there is 1 cup, grated yam

Switch to 'S' blade and process:

1 cup grated yam
1 cup sunflower seeds
1/4 cup soaked almonds
1/2 cup chopped celery
2 T. raisins, soaked 20 min. in 2 T. water (use all the water and raisins)
1 t. herbal seasoning
1 1/2 t. dried oregano
1 1/2 t. Veg-It

Form into 4 patties, about 1/4 to 1/2" thick. Place on oiled, solid dehydrator sheet and dehydrate 8-12 hours or until desired texture is acquired. Turn over after the first 6 hours and place on plastic mesh tray.

Sprouted Lentil Patties

In a food processor using the 'S' blade, process the following:

1 1/2 cups sprouted sunflower seeds
1 cup sprouted lentils
3 carrots, finely grated
1/2 white onion, chopped
3 stalks celery, chopped
2 garlic cloves, chopped
3 T. chopped parsley
1/2 inch slice of jalapeño pepper
3 T. lemon juice
2 t. poultry seasoning
1 t. tamari sauce
1/2 t. cumin
1 t. All Purpose seasoning

Form into patties about 1/2" thick and place on solid dehydrator sheet. Dehydrate 9-12 hours, changing to a mesh tray after 4 or 5 hours. Serve warm or cold.

Lani's Unfatty Sun Patties

Mix the following ingredients in a bowl and form into patties:

1 cup ground sunflower seeds (to a powder)
1/2 cup grated carrot
1/2 cup finely diced celery
2 thinly sliced green onions
1 T. chopped parsley
2 T. diced green bell pepper
2 T. diced red bell pepper
1/4 cup tomato juice (from fresh tomato)
1 T. olive oil or tahini
1/2 t. chili powder
1/2 t. sea salt
1/2 t. dried basil or 2 T. fresh basil
(if it needs more liquid, add some grated zucchini and 1 T. lemon juice)

Dehydrate on solid sheet until texture is right for you - crisp on outside, moist on inside. Flip over onto mesh sheet halfway through dehydrating time.

Variation: Add 1/2 cup of finely grated cabbage.

Tip: Any patty can be shaped into hot dog form instead of patty. Or patties can be shaped in flat, oval form. Whether dehydrated or not, they can be put in a Super Sushi Roll or Romaine lettuce leaf, rolled up and eaten as is or sliced into 2" slices.

Loaves

My Vegetable Nut Loaf

In a food processor, process the following using 'S' blade:

2 cups grated carrots
2 cups grated onions
2 cups sliced celery
2 cups walnuts, chopped
1 cup sunflower seeds
2 minced garlic cloves
2 T. tamari sauce

Form into loaf. Eat as is or dehydrate a few hours or until crisp on outside and moist on inside.

Serve on a lettuce-lined platter surrounded with grated beet and shredded green and red cabbage. Have your favorite sauce to spoon over.

Main Dishes

Lasagna

mixed summer squash, sliced and quartered (zucchini, button, yellow crookneck
tomatoes, chopped or cut in 1/2" chunks
Dressing: 1/4 cup olive oil
2 t. tamari sauce
fresh basil to taste
dried oregano, thyme
1 T. paprika
1/4 t. cayenne or chili powder
dill weed (optional) to taste

Mix dressing and pour over squash and tomatoes. Layer veggie mixture with sunflower seed cheese. Serve and enjoy.

Saturday Nite Chop Suey

1 sliced green onion
4 chopped mushrooms (if using dried shitake, soak for 30 min. in 1/4 to 1/2 cup water)
1 stalk of celery, sliced diagonally
1 bunch baby bok choy, sliced diagonally (leaves included)
4-5 sugar snap peas or Chines pea pods
1/2 bunch of Romaine lettuce - shredded or sliced thinly
3-4 red radishes, sliced thin
1 T. tamari sauce
1/2 cup mixed sprouts
dash of chili powder
dash of cayenne
4 cups loosely-packed mung bean sprouts

Mix together and spoon over the 4 cups of mung bean sprouts. Optional: 1/2 cup button mushrooms

Sauce: To soak water from shitake, mix in dash cayenne, 1 t. fresh grated ginger, 1/2 t. kelp powder, 1 T. celery powder or All Purpose Seasoning, 1 finely chopped green onion top, 4 more soaked shitake mushrooms, sliced thinly, 1 T. tamari sauce, 1 T. sesame oil and 1 ripe avocado. Mix thoroughly and pour over chop suey.

Eat with chopsticks. Make up fortunes.

Variation: Mix all together and serve as a pasta with fresh chopped tomatoes and cilantro on top. Omit the sauce.

Buckwheat Frisbee Pizza

Rub olive oil over top of Buckwheat Frisbees.
Sprinkle or spray aminos or tamari sauce on Frisbees.
Sprinkle on onion powder, cayenne and garlic powder, Italian seasoning, paprika, fresh or dried basil.
Place sun-dried tomatoes on top
Add slices of jicama, zucchini, mushrooms, olives, red pepper, green onion tops, thin-sliced red onion, avocado slices.
Sprinkle with olive oil and eat. Or sprinkle Sunrise Sauce flakes over all and eat.

Thin Pasta

Use a spiral slicer to make thin pasta out of:
zucchini, cucumber, beets, carrots, yams, butternut squash, yellow crookneck squash, sweet potatoes. Serve with your favorite dressing or sauce.
Add grated cabbage, mushrooms, etc. for a more colorful pasta..

Cheezy Cabbage Rolls

Mix 1 cup of your favorite seed cheese with the following:
some grated carrot
chopped red pepper
diced, drained cucumber
diced celery
garlic powder or granules
onion granules
finely chopped sweet onion
Bragg's aminos or tamari sauce

Pour hot water over several green cabbage leaves and soak for several seconds until wilted and pliable. Spoon 2-3 T. of above mixture into each leaf. Roll up, tucking ends under as you roll. Hold in place with a toothpick. Refrigerate. Serve on bed of lettuce with a dressing to dip the roll in. Eat with your hands. This makes a great finger food.

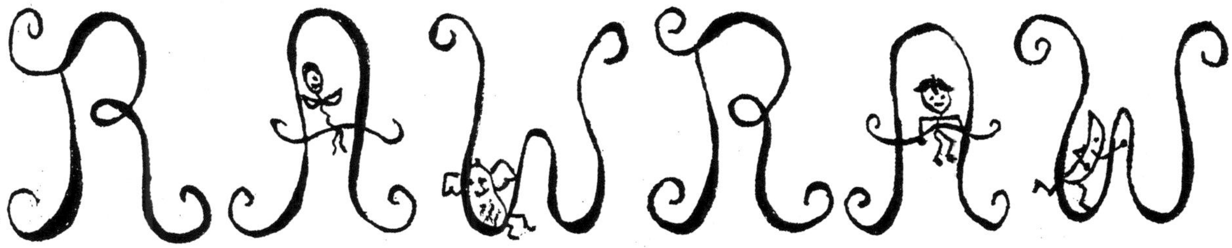

CHAPTER IX
SWEET SATISFACTIONS
(BALLS, COOKIES/BARS, CAKE, FROZEN DELIGHTS)

Energy Balls

Fudgie Balls (Fudgies)

In a bowl, mix with a spoon:

3/4 cup maple syrup
1 cup raw almond butter
1/2 cup raw walnuts, chopped coarsely
1/2 cup raw almonds, chopped coarsely
2-3 T. sunflower seeds
1/4 cup raw carob powder
1/3 cup Captain Buckwheat Crunch
1/4 cup unsweetened, shredded coconut
coconut - for rolling balls in

Refrigerate to harden. Form into walnut-size balls. Roll in shredded coconut. Freeze until ready to eat.

Variation: Substitute raw cashew butter for almond butter. Save in freezer and remove one or two at a time for an instant sweet sensation.

Marbles

3/4 cup raw almonds
1/2 cup raw tahini
3 T. honey
1 t. vanilla extract
2 T. plus 1 t. raw carob powder
Aphrodisiac Syrup

In food processor with 'S' blade, grind almonds well. Add tahini, honey, vanilla and mix well. Put half the mixture on a sheet of plastic wrap and press out into a square about 1/4 inch thick. To the rest of the dough, add carob powder and mix well. Press this mixture out on another piece of plastic wrap and press out to approximately the same dimensions. Wrap each mixture tightly and refrigerate for at least 1 hour. Unwrap each 'square'.

Carefully place the carob 'square' on top of the plain 'square'. Cut into small 1" squares. Roll each small square carefully between your palms to form a ball, marble-izing, but not completely mixing the two doughs. You want a contrast and marble of the carob vs. the plain dough. Freeze or refrigerate the balls in a covered plastic container.

Variation: add 1/2 t. cinnamon to plain dough after removing half the dough.

Variation: Before placing the carob 'square' on top of the plain 'square' spread plain square with a little Carob Aphrodisiac Syrup. Place carob 'square' on top of syrup and refrigerate. Instead of rolling into balls, cut into bars.

Choco Raisin Cashew Chews

This recipe was created when I was in a hurry and didn't have time to measure. I knew I couldn't go wrong.

tahini - I used over a cup
honey - about 3 T.
carob powder - about 1-2 T.
vanilla - 1 t.
raisins - a large handful (and then a few more)
cashews, chopped (about 1/2 cup)

Mix all together in a bowl. If too thin or moist, add more carob powder or raisins. Just play with the proportions, and be sure to taste each recipe entry until it suits you. It will taste delicious. Roll into small balls. I always refrigerate these chews, to hold their shape. Enjoy!

Tip: If you don't dry your own fruit, look for dried fruit that does not have sulphur dioxide added.

Carob Aphrodisiac Syrup

1/2 cup raw carob powder
1 cup maple syrup
1/4 cup olive oil
2 t. vanilla extract
1 T. raisins or dates
1/8 t. cinnamon

Mix all together in a bowl until smooth and well blended. Pour into covered bottle and store in the refrigerator. Can be eaten plain, whenever a craving for a sweet or chocolate takes over. Can drizzle over any bar (see Marbles), cookie or ball; or balls can be dipped into a small bowl of sauce. Use your imagination!

Raisin Chews

Powder 1/4 cup sesame seeds.

Add:

1 T. carob powder plus a little water
Mash in 1 handful of raisins
Add 1 handful sunflower seeds.

Form into balls. Chill.

Make Your Own Nut/Seed Balls

Mix combinations of the following:

Seeds: poppy, pumpkin, sunflower, sesame, or flax (ground or whole)
Nuts: almonds, Brazil, walnuts, coconut, pecans, cashew, macadamias or filberts (ground or chopped)

Add:

Dried fruit: apple, Black Mission figs, Calimyrna figs, dried plums, raisins, currants, dates, apricots, peaches, pineapple, bananas, papaya, mango, cherries, pears

Process using 'S' blade after nuts are chopped or ground and seeds are chopped or ground.

Mix in any raw nut butter: almond, tahini, cashew

Add raw carob powder if desired for 'chocolate' flavor or cinnamon.

Add a sweetener if desired: honey, barley malt or pure maple syrup, vanilla extract.

Form into balls and refrigerate.

Variation: Can roll balls in finely ground nuts or unsweetened coconut powdered to look like powdered 'sugar'. I like to add pumpkin and sunflower seeds whole into the bowl of nut butter, carob and maple syrup. Very simple, crunchy and satisfying.

Tahini Balls

You create. Mix 2 T. tahini, 1/2 cup sunflower seed sprouts or sunflower seeds, ground, 2 T. carob powder, 2-3 T. maple syrup, dried coconut to make thick and chopped cashews, or your favorite nut. Play with the ingredients until it satisfies your taste for a sweet treat. Roll in balls and roll in Almond-Cinnamon Mixture, sesame seeds or ground nuts. Freeze and eat when in need of a sweet treat.

Variation: Use less maple syrup and add a small handful of raisins, 1 t. carob powder and some macadamia nuts in place of cashews.

Cookies/Energy Bars

Fluffy, White Clouds (A Light Cookie with a Thousand Variations)

In a food processor, using the 'S' blade:

1 cup sprouted sunflower seeds (sprouted 1 or 2 days after soaking overnight)
1 cup sprouted almonds - soak overnight, rinse, then sprout for half-a-day
14-16 dates - not the large Medjool - use the California dates that are smaller. Be sure to slice open each date and remove the pit.
1 peeled banana
1 t. almond extract

Process until well-mixed, but still chunky. Do not make a smooth dough out of this mixture. You want some chunky dates, banana, nuts and seeds.

In a blender, pour in:

1/2 cup unsweetened coconut (shredded or flaked)

Blend until the coconut is as fine as powdered sugar. Pour into a small bowl.

Roll small walnut-size balls of dough between your hands, then roll in the coconut and place 1 1/2" apart on a solid dehydrator sheet. Taking a tamper or bottom of a glass, flatten each 'cloud' to a height of 1/2 inch.

Dehydrate at around 100 degrees approximately 4 hours; using a spatula, turn cookies over onto a mesh sheet and dehydrate for about 3-5 hours or until firm on outside and moist on the inside. These cookies are so light, you can eat and enjoy them, knowing there is no sugar, artificial fat or additives. Yummy! Makes about 1 1/2 dozen.

Variations: For those who don't like coconut, you can powder 1/2 cup raw cashews, turning them into flour for rolling the mixture in.

You can replace the banana with apple chunks and add a dash of cinnamon, use soaked raisins in place of dates, walnuts in place of almonds and 1 t. vanilla extract rather than almond. Roll in coarsely ground pecans or walnuts.

You can use sesame seeds in place of sunflower seeds. Just coarsely grind with a mortar and pestle, or use flax seed soaked or ground. Your choice

Try dried apricots, fresh blueberries This could be a cookie with no exact measurements, just your taste buds directing your creative imagination to create a cookie from whatever you have available.

Super Flax Cookie

In food processor, using 'S' blade, pulse chop the following ingredients:

2 T. maple syrup
1/2 t. cinnamon
a small handful of walnut halves
1 small apple, cored and cut into wedges

Stir in 1/4 cup soaked flax seeds (no water left in flax-but will be gelatinous)

Form round, 1/4" thick, cookie shape on solid dehydrator sheet and dry below 100 degrees for a few hours, transferring to a mesh. Continue to dehydrate until outside is crisp and inside chewy and soft, approximately a total of 12 hours. Makes 1 large or 2 cookies.

Sprout Cookies

In food processor, using 'S' blade, process until smooth the following:

1 cup sprouted soft wheatberries
1/3 cup soaked cashews
1/2 t. vanilla extract

Add:

1/4 cup unsweetened, shredded coconut
3 T. carob powder
1/4 cup raisins (heaping)

Pulse the mixture with the added coconut, carob and raisins.

Roll into walnut size balls, flatten with bottom of glass to make round cookies and dehydrate on solid sheet until crisp on outside and chewy inside. Flip onto mesh sheet after a few hours of dehydrating.

ABC Cookies (apple-buckwheat-cashew)

In food processor, using 'S' blade, chop
1 cup sprouted wheatberries
Add:
1/2 apple, unpeeled and sliced
1/4 cup raw cashew nuts
2/3 cup soaked raisins
1 T. flax seed, ground
Chop or pulse several times. Then stir in:
1 t. almond extract
1/4 cup finely chopped almonds
3 T. Captain Buckwheat Crunch.

Form into balls, flatten on solid dehydrator tray and dehydrate at 95-100 degrees until crisp on outside and chewy inside.

High Protein Sesame Seed Energy Bars

cashew butter or almond butter
sesame seeds, hulled, unbleached
sunflower seeds
pumpkin seeds
unsweetened coconut flakes or shreds
honey
sea salt
vanilla extract

Mix these ingredients up with a spoon in a bowl, according to your taste. Begin with some cashew butter. Sesame seeds should predominate, with enough other seeds and coconut to make a stiff mixture. Taste and adjust ingredients until you are satisfied. You can never make too many, so if you have to add more cashew butter or more seeds or coconut, it's okay. These will last a long time, wrapped and refrigerated. Press mixture (about 1/2-3/4" thick) into oiled glass pan. Refrigerate to harden. Then cut into 2" squares.

Cake

Not Just Any Carrot Cake

In a food processor, using the 'S' blade, process the following:

4 cups grated carrots
1 cup almonds, soaked overnight and peeled
1 cup dates, pitted

Transfer to a bowl. Mix remaining ingredients well with carrot-nut-date mixture.

1 cup raisins
3/4 cup walnuts, soaked 4-5 hours, chopped
3/4 cup shredded coconut
2 T. flax seeds, ground
2 t. vanilla extract
1/4 t. cinnamon

Press firmly into a pie plate. Refrigerate at least one hour.

Frosting: In a food processor, using 'S' attachment, process the following:

1 cup dates, pitted
1/2 cup pine nuts
1/2 cup raw macadamia or cashew nuts
1/2 cup orange juice
1 t. vanilla or almond extract
1 t. orange zest

Can try to blend in blender until light and fluffy.

Then dollop over the cake or spread the frosting over the cake and serve. Looks great decorated with green and red grapes, sliced kiwi fruit, tangerine boats. Stand kiwi or tangerine slices up along sides of cake, making a dent with a spoon along the edges for each kiwi slice or tangerine boat.

Frozen Desserts

Mango Freeze

1-2 cups mango chunks, frozen
1/3 cup almond milk

Puree in blender until creamy.
Spoon into parfait glasses.

Smoothies to Eat

1 cup frozen peaches, apricots, plums or nectarines (or mangos or papaya)
1 frozen banana
1/2 cup fresh orange juice or apple juice

Chop in food processor or blender, then blend until smooth.
Serve immediately in small goblets.

Strawberry-Banana Sherbet

2 bananas
8-10 strawberries
2-3 T. lemon juice

Blend bananas and strawberries together in blender together with a little lemon juice; freeze in ice cube tray. When frozen, put cubes into blender and blend just until sherbet consistency. Serve immediately.

Variations: Use any fruit or fruit combinations, along with 2-3 T. lemon juice. Puree in blender, freeze in shallow trays or ice cube trays. When ready to serve, blend until of sherbet consistency and eat.

Tip: For a sorbet, freeze fresh juices in ice cube trays, then put through inexpensive snow cone hand-cranked machine for shaved ice. Or put through blank plate on your Champion juicer.

Fruit Sherbets

Choose from a variety of fresh fruits (bananas, cherries, nectarines, peaches, strawberries).

Freeze the fruit - either whole, sliced or pureed (if pureed, pour into ice cube trays).

When solid, put a just little fruit juice into the blender (apple, orange, grape, lemon, pineapple), add the frozen fruit chunks or cubes and blend until mixture is of sherbet consistency. Only add as much juice as you need to get it mixed smoothly.

What? No Dairy, Ice Cream

Freeze banana chunks.

In a blender, pour about one cup very cold nut or seed milk. Add almond, maple or vanilla extract to flavor. Or add carob powder or finely chopped nuts.

Add frozen banana chunks and blend everything until of ice cream consistency. Add more banana chunks if necessary. Eat immediately or freeze until it hardens back up.

Dessert in a Melon

papaya or melon
strawberry-banana sherbet
sunflower seed sprouts
cinnamon

Cut papaya or melon in half and scoop out seeds. Fill center with sherbet, then garnish with sprouts and cinnamon.

Cool Sundaes or Banana Split

1. For banana split, slice a banana in half lengthwise and place on plate. For sundae, get a large bowl.
2. Place 3 scoops of sherbet, no-dairy ice cream or other flavors onto plate or bowl.
3. Fruit: Spoon fresh, sliced fruit around the ice cream or sherbet - peaches, bananas, melon balls, berries
4. Sauce: Spoon or drizzle over any or all three of the following: carob sauce, maple syrup, fruit puree
5. Topping: dried fruit, diced dates, raisins, apricots, apples
6. Nuts: finely chopped walnuts, almonds, pecans, cashews, macadamia nuts
7. More: sunflower seeds, Captain Buckwheat Crunch, cinnamon, shredded coconut
8. Settle back with a spoon, eat and enjoy.

Banana Ice Cream

In a blender, blend 2 frozen bananas cut into chunks. Serve immediately.

Frozen Banana Pops

Cut peeled bananas in half. Insert popsicle sticks in wide end of banana halves. Roll in carob powder and honey mixture. Roll in almond meal or sunflower seed meal. Freeze.

Variation: Roll banana in thick 'Chocolate' Sauce and then shredded coconut and freeze.

Thick 'Chocolate' Sauce

1/2 cup soaked cashews or pecans
1/4 cup pitted dates
1/4 cup raisins
1-3 T. carob powder
1/4 cup almond milk

Blend all ingredients to make a thick sauce.

Variation: Make sauce to dip apple slices in or banana slices.

Variation: For fudge, mix in 1 T. ground flax seed and 1-2 T. chopped walnuts. Spread in shallow dish and refrigerate or freeze. Cut into small squares. Alternative: Roll in balls and freeze.

RAW RAW

CHAPTER X
TEN WEEKS OF LIVE FOOD MENUS

Below are the meals I ate for the first five weeks of my ten-week eating plan. I decided to go cold turkey eating raw, living foods. Everyday after work, I would browse through my raw food books to find some recipes to try out. I was very busy the first week. I tried everything. In the first week, I prepared 21 different recipes and sprouted 8 grains, seeds or nuts. It was very exciting and exhausting. I also increased my exercise program. After all, it was the beginning of a New Year. I was on a fitness team with points given for exercise and pounds lost. I had support. You can ask a friend to be your support buddy, even if this friend is on a different eating plan, or doesn't need to lose weight, but wants to increase his/her exercise.

Hopefully, you will find ideas of what you can eat by reading what I ate and browsing through the recipes. Feel free to simplify and vary the menu items, especially if you are beginning this program in a different season, when different fruits and vegetables are grown and harvested. You will soon be able to use those fruits and vegetables in similar recipes. You will adapt. Recipes are included in this book for the items that are capitalized.

Keep in mind that I began my diet on New Year's Day, so most of my foods are what were in season locally during the winter. If you decide to begin during spring, summer or fall, you will most likely be purchasing primarily local foods in season. Summertime is relatively easy because there are so many fresh fruits, greens and salad vegetables available. Think of all the salsas you can make for toppings or dips, using fresh onions and tomatoes. Delicious pears, peaches, apricots, and many other fruits are available at a good price. Keep in mind that many of my ingredients in shakes, juices and green salads are interchangeable with many summertime ingredients, or spring or fall, for that matter. Be creative and create your own beautiful fruit and vegetable salads.

My Food and Exercise Log

Week 1.

Day 1 exercise - walk a treadmill

Breakfast: Power Smoothie (4 carrots, juiced, 2 oranges juiced, 1 green lettuce leaf, 1 T. flax seeds, ground, 1/2 frozen banana-all put in blender and blended until smooth.)

Snack: 0

Lunch: My Big Basic Salad Bowl - (Mixed greens, shredded purple cabbage, clover sprouts, mixture of mung and lentil sprouts, baby carrots, dollop of Oregon Hummus, green onion, 1/3 of avocado, sliced, nori strips, a small handful of almond-walnut-sunflower seed mixture) Dressing: 2-3 T. miso dressing.

Snack: herb tea, two Pecan-Date Balls, 3-4 raw almonds

Dinner: 1 apple, sliced, 1 kiwi fruit, peeled and sliced

Day 2 exercise - walk, yoga

Breakfast: Power Smoothie

Snack: carob/nut/seed square, herb tea

Lunch: My Big Basic Salad Bowl Same as Day 1.

Snack: a few almonds, 1 tiny Tahini Ball, 1 small sunflower seed cookie

Dinner: Veggie-Nut Patty with a small green salad, avocado slices

Snack: 2 small Marbles, 1 Medjool date, 1/2 banana

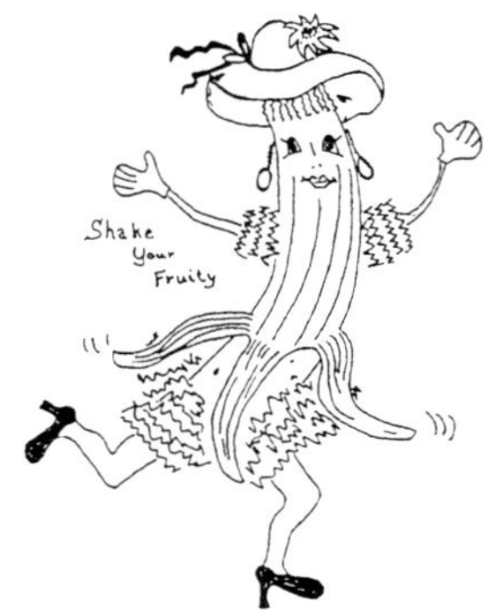

Day 3 exercise - cardio/wts.

Breakfast: Liquid Sunshine

Snack: 1 black olive

Lunch: Broccoli-In-Bed, Sunrise Sauce, Veggie-Nut Patty with miso dressing

Snack: 0

Dinner: 2 kiwi, sliced; 1 Fluffy White Cloud Cookie, 1/2 banana, a few walnuts

Day 4 exercise - step aerobics

Breakfast: Power Smoothie

Snack: 1 Fluffy White Cloud Cookie

Lunch: Heavenly Salad, Veggie-Nut Patty, with Sunrise Sauce

Snack: 1 T. Carob Aphrodisiac Syrup, 1 Medjool date

Dinner: 2 kiwi fruit, sliced, 1 apple sliced, 1/2 banana sliced, 1/4 t. cinnamon, sprinkled over the fruit

Day 5 exercise - none
Breakfast: Liquid Sunshine
Snack: 0
Lunch: My Big Basic Salad Bowl (with mixed greens, grated carrots, cucumber sticks, sliced yellow squash, purple cabbage, celery, diced, a few walnuts, 2 Brazil nuts) miso dressing, sprinkled with dehydrated Sunrise Sauce (flakes)
Snack: Miso Soup with raw peas, grated carrot, sliced green onions (lukewarm)
Dinner: 1 kiwi, sliced

Day 6 exercise - yoga, step aerobics
Breakfast: Whole Grain Cereal
Snack: water
Lunch: My Big Basic Salad Bowl, Spicy Jicama 'Stix'
Snack: water
Dinner: peppermint tea, dried fruit (mixture), raw nut mix (almonds, pecans, walnuts)

Day 7 yoga
Breakfast: Whole Grain Cereal (with soaked raisins, sprouted sunflower seeds and a dash of cinnamon), fresh orange juice
Snack: several mixed raw nuts
Lunch: Heavenly Salad
Snack: 1 Fluffy White Cloud Cookie
Dinner: 1 apple and 1 kiwi
Snack: 2 Marbles, 1 t. Carob Aphrodisiac Syrup

Tip: After the third or fourth day I stopped craving junk sweets. The fresh fruit and salads were helping me to kick the sugar habit. I also cut caffeine cold turkey but wouldn't advise it if you've been dependent on coffee to get you going each morning or soft drinks. Since I usually had a decaf. mocha, I wasn't addicted to caffeine, just the sugar. So, you might have a withdrawal headache if you quit coffee cold. Just decrease gradually until you wean yourself. Find an herbal tea substitute that is spicy and tasty, hearty, like a cup of coffee, but without the caffeine.

Week 2

Day 1 walk, weights

Breakfast: Liquid Sunshine

Lunch: small glass of lemon juice and water, 1 Sprouted Lentil Patty drizzled with olive oil, My Big Basic Salad Bowl, 3 T. Curried Lentil-Mung-Adzuki Sprout Salad

Snack: 2 High Protein Sesame Seed Energy Bars, 1 T. flax oil

Dinner: 3 T. Oregon Hummus with dehydrated sweet potato 'chips', Flax Crackers

Day 2 step aerobics

Breakfast: Power Smoothie

Lunch: My Big Basic Salad Bowl, Curried Lentil-Mung-Adzuki Sprout Salad, 2 Sprouted Lentil Patties

Snack: 1 apple

Dinner: 1 large carrot, sliced diagonally into slices. Large dollop of Oregon Hummus, 1/4 of an avocado, sliced

Day 3 body pump

Breakfast: Power Smoothie

Snack: 1 shot of wheat grass juice, High Protein Sesame Seed Energy Bar, herbal tea

Lunch: 1 handful raw cashew nuts, 1 Asian pear

Dinner: My Big Basic Salad Bowl

Day 4 walking

Breakfast: Power Smoothie

Lunch: 1 Asian pear, 2 High Protein Sesame Seed Energy Bars, 1 cup of veggie slices (red onion rings, zucchini rounds, cucumber sticks and carrot circles with a miso dressing (white miso, safflower oil, cider vinegar, lemon juice, shoyu, chopped yellow onion, blended smooth)

Dinner: My Big Basic Salad Bowl, 1/2 cup Curried Lentil-Mung-Adzuki Sprout Salad, Oregon Hummus, carrot slices

Day 5 walking

Breakfast: Power Smoothie

Lunch: 2 Sprouted Lentil Patties with miso dressing, 1 Asian pear

Snack: 2 T. almond butter with a little honey, sesame seeds and sunflower seed sprouts

Dinner: My Big Basic Salad Bowl, Curried Lentil-Mung-Adzuki Sprout Salad, Oregon Hummus as dressing

Snack 1 t. Carob Aphrodisiac Syrup

Day 6 clogging

Breakfast: Power Smoothie

Lunch: 2 Sprouted Lentil Patties with Oregon Hummus and avocado slices

Snack: 10 oz. carrot juice, carrots juiced with 3 kale leaves

Dinner: 1/4 of a mango, sliced

Day 7 yoga
Breakfast: Power Smoothie
Lunch: Oregon Hummus set in bowl in center of plate. Surrounding bowl were dark green lettuce leaves, alfalfa sprouts, sliced radishes, avocado slices, 2 green onions, Curried Lentil-Mung-Adzuki Sprout Salad. Hooked on edge of the hummus bowl were strips of sweet red pepper. In front part of plate were sweet potato 'chips' and Crunchy Sweet Flax Crackers
Snack: 4 oz. carrot juice
Dinner: Oregon Hummus roll-ups - Place a dollop of hummus in center of large Romaine or red leaf lettuce leaf, add strip of red pepper, avocado slice and a squirt of miso dressing. Roll up like a burrito and eat with hands. 2 Sprouted Lentil Patties
Snack: 2 High Protein Sesame Seed Energy Bars

Week 3
Day 1 step aerobics
Breakfast: Power Smoothie
Snack: 4 oz. carrot juice
Lunch: My Big Basic Salad Bowl, 2 Sprouted Lentil Patties, 1 Yummy Yammy Patty
Snack: 6 oz. carrot juice, 1 High Protein Sesame Seed Energy Bar
Dinner: 1 Yummy Yammy Patty on salad greens and sprouts with miso dressing, 1 small bowl mango
Snack: a few nuts - walnuts and pecans, 3-4 dates stuffed with pecans, lemon-zinger herbal tea

Day 2 yoga
Breakfast: 1 small bowl sprouted soft-wheat blended just a little with raisins and cinnamon
Snack: water
Lunch: Power Smoothie with 2 kale leaves
Snack: fresh juiced orange, 1 High Protein Sesame Seed Energy Bars
Dinner: small dinner salad with mixed greens, sprouts, avocado, sliced red pepper and grated carrots, 1 Super Sushi Roll using crumbled Yummy Yammy Patty as filling with sunflower seeds, carrot, gr. onion and red pepper strips.
Snack: 1 whole ruby red grapefruit

Day 3 cardio/wts., dance
Breakfast: Power Smoothie
Snack: water
Lunch: 1 apple
Snack: 1 cup warm herbal tea
Dinner: green salad with cilantro, grated cabbage, carrots, green onions, 1 Super Sushi Roll using crumbled Yummy Yammy Patty as filling
Snack: 2 lettuce leaves, 1/2 small avocado, 1 T. raw tahini, 1 ruby red grapefruit

Day 4 step aerobics
Breakfast: Power Smoothie
Snack: water
Lunch: 1 Super Sushi Roll using Party Pate' as filling with avocado, red pepper strips, carrot matchsticks, green onion strips on top, a few squirts of miso dressing and alfalfa sprouts at end of rolling up
Snack: 1 t. Carob Aphrodisiac Syrup
Dinner: 3-4 Fudgies (Fudgie Balls)

Day 5 no exercise
Breakfast: 1 bowl of sprouted wheat/kamut/spelt/raisin cookie (dehydrated)
Power Smoothie, 1 Fudgie
Snack: 2 Fudgie Balls, 1 sprouted wheat/kamut/spelt/raisin cookie
Lunch: 1 Super Sushi Roll
Snack: 1 apple
Dinner: fruit salad using 1/2 mango, sliced; kiwi slices, one-half banana, sliced with cinnamon sprinkled on top
Snack: water

Day 6 yoga, wts., clogging
Breakfast: 4 mini-slices of sprouted wheat/kamut/spelt bread (about 1" high) with 1 t. flax oil sprinkled over the top; 1 cup warm herbal tea
Snack: 1 slice dried papaya (no sulphur dioxide), 4 filberts
Lunch: My Big Basic Salad Bowl using clover sprouts and adding shredded broccoli-cabbage-carrot mixture (store-bought), 1/3 avocado, sliced and a handful of mixed raw nuts and seeds, with miso dressing
Snack: 1 Fudgie Ball
Dinner: 1 ruby red grapefruit

Day 7 yoga, weights
Breakfast: 3 thin slices sprouted wheat/kamut/spelt/raisin bread with flax oil sprinkled over the top
Snack: water
Lunch: My Big Basic Salad Bowl - with Curried Lent-Mung-Adzuki Sprout Salad on top along with the broccoli-cabbage-carrot mixture (store-bought). bowl of Party Pate' with cucumber circles, mini carrots and radish slices to dip into the pate'
Snack: 3 Fudgie Balls, water
Dinner: ruby red grapefruit
Snack: pieces of the sprouted wheat/kamut/spelt/raisin bread with flax oil on top

Tip: Plan your menus a few days ahead so you will know when to soak your seeds or grains or nuts to sprout for the recipes coming up.

Week 4

Day 1 cardio/wts.
Breakfast: Power Smoothie, adding 2 kale leaves, 2-3 T. sunflower seeds and 1 T. nutritional yeast
Snack: water
Lunch: My Big Basic Salad Bowl with Curried Lentil-Mung-Adzuki Sprout Salad on top, a side bowl of avocado slices, mini-carrots and cucumber circles to dip into a big dollop of Party Pate', 1 bowl of Broccoli-In-Bed with Sunrise Sauce
Snack: 2 Fudgie Balls
Dinner: 1 kiwi, sliced, apple slices

Day 2 yoga, weights
Breakfast: Power Smoothie
Snack: a few nuts and sprouted sunflower seeds
Lunch: zucchini, butternut squash noodles with miso dressing
Snack: 1 apple
Dinner: 1 ruby red grapefruit

Day 3 cardio/wts.
Breakfast: Power Smoothie
Snack: some carrot sticks with Party Pate'
Lunch: Heavenly Salad, Veggie-Nut Patty
Snack: 1 apple, 2 stalks celery
Dinner: Veggie-Nut Patty with Sunrise Sauce
Snack: 1 Tahini Ball, sprouted wheat/kamut/spelt/raisin bread, sliced with flax oil

Day 4 step aerobics
Breakfast: Power Smoothie
Snack: water
Lunch: My Big Basic Salad Bowl with Sunrise Sauce dressing and Broccoli-In-Bed
Snack: some carrot sticks with Party Pate'
Dinner: 1 ruby red grapefruit

Day 5 walk
Breakfast: Power Smoothie
Snack: water
Lunch: Bowl of yellow crookneck "spaghetti" topped with Sunrise Sauce, with Curried Lentil-Mung-Adzuki Sprout Salad on the side, 1/2 avocado with clover sprouts over all. A bowl full of Spicy Jicama 'Stix' sprinkled with paprika and onion powder
Snack: 5 Fudgie Balls
Dinner: ruby red grapefruit
Snack: 2 pieces Sprouted Wheat, Raisin, Cinnamon Bread with raw almond butter and sliced bananas

Day 6 clogging
Breakfast: Detox Tea
Snack: water
Lunch: mixed greens, red onion, grated raw beet, peas, zucchini cubes, celery, miso dressing
Snack: raw cookie with flax seed, walnuts and blueberries
Dinner: ruby red grapefruit

Day 7 yoga
Breakfast: Detox tea
Snack: water
Lunch: apple
Snack: My Big Basic Salad Bowl with shredded broccoli-cabbage-carrot slaw, Curried Lentil-Mung-Adzuki Sprout Salad, 1/2 avocado, Mi Miso Dressing, dollop of Sunrise Sauce on top. 4 baby carrots, red onion, purple cabbage
Dinner: ruby red grapefruit
Snack: 2 ABC Cookies

Week 5
Day 1 step aerobics, weights
Breakfast: Detox tea
Snack: water
Lunch: plate of mixed greens with 3 mini carrots, Cauliflower Mash (Green), with 1 t. flax oil and paprika, Quinoa Tabouleh, Tuna-4-2 Salad in 1/4 of a red pepper cup, surrounded by clover sprouts and avocado slices
Snack: 1 ABC Cookie
Dinner: ruby red grapefruit
Snack: 1 Super Flax Cookie, 1 Sprouted Lentil Patty

Day 2 yoga
Breakfast: 1 Sprouted Lentil Patty, Power Smoothie with 1 T. flax seeds, ground, 3 kale leaves, protein powder, 1 t. calcium citrate, 1 T. nutritional yeast, banana and blueberries, 1 Super Flax Cookie
Snack: 1 ABC Cookie, 1 small, Crisp Buckwheat Frisbee, 1 with miso dressing spread on it and Tuna-2 with sprouts, 1 with Cauliflower Mash (Green) spread on it with avocado slices on top
Lunch: a plate of greens and sprouts with Quinoa Tabouleh, Tuna-4-2 in red pepper cup, Cauliflower Mash (Green) with 1 t. flax oil
Snack: 2 Fluffy White Cloud Cookies, 1 ABC Cookie
Dinner: water
Snack: 1 Fluffy White Cloud Cookie

Day 3 cardio, weights
Breakfast: 1 small glass grape juice
Snack: 2 Fluffy White Cloud Cookies
Lunch: plate of greens and clover sprouts with serving of Quinoa Tabouleh, a big dollop of Cauliflower Mash with 1 t. flax oil, and some red bell pepper strips with Tuna-4-2, 4 mini-carrots and slices of avocado, 2 T. Sunrise Sauce, 1 small Sprouted Lentil Patty, Mi Miso Dressing over salad
Snack: 1 Fluffy White Cloud Cookie, 1 Fudgie Ball rolled in coconut, 1 whole Asian pear
Dinner: 2 Crisp Buckwheat Frisbees - one spread with mashed avocado and sprinkled with kelp, the other spread with Mi Miso Dressing and diced tomatoes. Very tasty and filling.
Snack: 0

Day 4 walk
Breakfast: glass of grape juice
Snack: 0
Lunch: Power Smoothie (with 2 kale leaves, 1 T. sunflower seeds, 1 T. nutritional yeast, 1 T. spirulina, 1 scoop green protein powder, 1 T. flax seeds, ground, 3 oranges, juiced, 1/2 frozen banana, 1/4 cup blueberries)
Snack: 1 Fudgie Ball rolled in coconut
Dinner: My Big Basic Salad Bowl with Quinoa Tabouleh, Tuna-4-2, parsley, red pepper, red cabbage, mung bean sprouts, carrots, avocado, cucumber, diced white onion,
Snack: 1 Fluffy White Cloud Cookie, 1 Fudgie Ball

Day 5 no exercise
Breakfast: grape juice
Snack: 0
Lunch: 2 big strawberries, 2/3 of a banana
Snack: 2 oz. wheat grass juice with lime juice
Dinner: Mixed greens, red cabbage, sprouts, Tuna-4-2, Cauliflower Mash with 1 t. flax oil, 5 mini carrots, 4 cucumber slices, a little red pepper, 2/3 of an avocado, sliced, miso dressing, parsley sprigs
Snack: 2 Fudgie Balls

Day 6 clogging
Breakfast: grape juice
Snack: Power Smoothie
Lunch: small helping Cauliflower Mash with 1 t. flax oil
Snack: 3 mini carrots, Miso 'Drink'
Dinner: My Big Basic Salad Bowl with clover sprouts on top, Mi Miso Dressing, 1/2 avocado, red cabbage, red pepper, cucumber slices and sprouted sunflower seeds.

Day 7 yoga
Breakfast: grape juice
Snack: 1 1/4" slice of Party Paté
Lunch: My Big Basic Salad Bowl - mixed greens, red leaf lettuce. Then Mi Miso Dressing poured on top, then shredded red cabbage, sunflower seed sprouts, 1/2 cup grated yam, clover sprouts; topped with a dollop of Cauliflower Mash with 1 t. flax oil. 4 cucumber slices on side, 1/2 avocado sliced around plate. 3 flax seed crackers for 3 1/4" slices of Party Paté. Very pretty - red, green, purple, orange
Snack: 1 Fudgie Ball
Dinner: 1 ruby red grapefruit
Snack: 0

Congratulations! You've just finished five weeks! Now, go out and buy yourself something sexy and fun to wear. When I completed my first 5 weeks I had lost 15 pounds and was feeling so light and healthy that I wanted to complete the next 5 weeks eating live foods only, also. I felt I could simplify a bit, now that I had created some fabulous - to look at and eat - meals. Most of the other recipes in this book were incorporated, discovered, created, prepared, after the final 5 weeks, into the next few months up to the present. By now, you will know how to modify your meals, too.

Remember, the only rule here is to eat a *variety* of fresh raw fruits and vegetables, a few soaked or sprouted nuts, seeds and grains. How you eat these is up to you. Just try to strike a balance between the sweet fruits, green leafy vegetables and fatty avocados, olives, coconut, nuts and seeds. You can do primarily shakes, juices and salads accompanied by patés, sauces, purees, and yogurt/seed cheeses, like I did, with dehydrated patties and crackers for variety in texture and taste. It's turned out to be easier than I thought and can be simplified.

As long as you don't add many cooked foods to the menu, you WILL lose weight!!

* *

I will provide the final 5 weeks of what I ate. However, I have discovered, finally, how really simple it is to prepare my foods and how I seem to require less food than I ever ate before. The food I eat is packed with vitamins and minerals, so my body seems to know what it needs. I eat more intuitively. If I feel like fruit for lunch and green salad for dinner, I have just that. If I feel like fruit for a day, I follow my intuition. Basically, it becomes very simple. Here is a typical day:

Breakfast: water and a piece of fruit
Snack: a piece of fruit, a few nuts
Lunch: Power Smoothie with various additions
Snack: sometimes a sweet seed/nut ball or piece of fruit
Dinner: My Big Basic Salad Bowl
Snack: grapefruit or dried fruit

In other words, I make sure I have several pieces of fruit a day, either plain, in a fruit salad or a shake or smoothie. I always have a big, green salad with sprouts, watery veggies, other grated or finely chopped veggies, sprouts, and a few sprouted or soaked beans, nuts, or seeds, plus avocado, *always*. When I feel like making it, I'll have a seed cheese or sauce to accompany my salad. I always make my own dressings. I nearly always have about 1/3 to 1 avocado daily (best with greens). I nearly always add a kale, collard or red Swiss chard leaf to my Power Smoothie for added minerals, including calcium.

I soak nuts 50% of the time. Adding almonds to a smoothie supplements the drink with magnesium. Water is my main drink, sometimes with lemon juice added to it. I don't have sweets every day, but when I do, it is often a nut/seed ball. I only eat dried fruit that is sun-dried with no sulphur dioxide added. I like to dehydrate fruit leathers, fruit for chewing on or for muesli, sliced veggies for chips and an occasional burger, loaf or bread.

Week 6
Day 1 step aerobics, weights
Breakfast: Power Smoothie
Snack: 0
Lunch: mixed spring greens, red leaf lettuce, sunflower seed sprouts with Mi Miso Dressing
4 mini carrots, 1 Yummy Yammy Patty, slice of Party Pate', 1/2 avocado
Snack: 2 Fudgies
Dinner: grapefruit
Snack: 1/2" slice Party Pate' plus 1 t. Mi Miso Dressing
1 Fudgie Ball

Day 2 yoga
Breakfast: 1 glass of Liver Detoxifying Drink
Snack: 1 glass of Liver Detoxifying Drink
Lunch: 1 glass of Liver Detoxifying Drink
Snack: 1 glass of Liver Detoxifying Drink
Dinner: 1 glass of Liver Detoxifying Drink
Snack: 1 glass of Liver Detoxifying Drink

Day 3 weights, step aerobics
Breakfast: 1 glass of Liver Detoxifying Drink
Snack: 1 kiwi, 1 banana, 1/2 mango, sliced into a bowl with cinnamon sprinkled
Lunch: My Big Basic Salad Bowl, 1 Yummy Yammy Patt y
Snack: herb tea, 2 Fudgies
Dinner: 0
Snack: 0

Day 4 yoga
Breakfast: 0
Snack: crumbled Yummy Yammy Patty with Mi Miso Dressing
Lunch: My Big Basic Salad Bowl with Mi Miso Dressing
Snack: 1/2 grapefruit, a few almonds and walnuts, some mini-carrots
Dinner: sliced tomatoes on greens with avocado-lemon juice dressing
Snack: 2 Fudgies, 3/4 of an apple

Day 5 no exercise
Breakfast: Power Smoothie
Snack: 0
Lunch: 0
Snack: big helping of Cauliflower Mash with 1 t. flax oil
Dinner: 4 Fudgie Balls
Snack: 0

Day 6 clogging
Breakfast: 1 banana
Snack: 0
Lunch: 8-9 almonds, a few sprouted sunflower seeds, 1 apple
Snack: My Big Basic Salad Bowl - red Swiss chard, chunks of yellow and zucchini squash, red and yellow peppers, red cabbage, 1/3 avocado with miso dressing, shot of wheat grass juice
Dinner: Cauliflower Mash with 1 t. flax oil
Snack: 1 big T. almond butter, chopped pecans, 2 t. maple syrup, 1/2 t. carob powder - mixed together

Day 7 yoga
Breakfast: 1/2 banana
Snack: 0
Lunch: rest of yesterday's salad, a few almonds and walnuts, 2 tangelos
Snack: avocado with Cauliflower Mash
Dinner: ugli fruit
Snack: a bunch of broken cashew nuts

Week 7
Day 1 no exercise
Breakfast: Power Smoothie
Snack: herb tea
Lunch: 1 tangerine, date-sunflower seed cookie (dehydrated), handful nuts and seeds, 6 strawberries, 2 Sprouted Lentil Patties
Snack: red pepper strips, zucchini, cucumbers
Dinner: My Big Basic Salad Bowl
Snack: 0

Day 2 walk, weights
Breakfast: 1 tangerine, 1 apple
Snack: herbal tea
Lunch: My Big Basic Salad Bowl, 3 date-sunflower seed cookies, some almonds and walnuts
Snack: 2 Fudgies, a handful of chopped cashews, 2 T. almond nut butter
Dinner: 1/2 mango
Snack: red grapefruit

Day 3 step aerobics, weights
Breakfast: 0
Snack: 0
Lunch: Power Smoothie with 3 kale leaves
Snack: 1/2 banana, some cashews, herbal tea
Dinner: My Big Basic Salad Bowl with some almonds and walnuts, sprouts, 1 avocado, grated carrots, cabbage, sliced tomatoes and cucumber and cubed jicama and a miso dressing
Snack: raw store-bought cookie, 1/2 orange

Day 4 walk
Breakfast: Power Smoothie
Snack: 1 pear, 1 tangerine, 1/2 avocado, herb tea
Lunch: small handful cashews
Snack: a few raw macadamia nuts and walnuts, slices of orange and grapefruit
Dinner: My Big Basic Salad Bowl with avocado, sugar snap peas, spinach-almond pesto, red pepper, and raw asparagus, sliced diagonally
Snack: 2 dates

Day 5 walk
Breakfast: Power Smoothie with frozen bananas and mixed berries
Snack: raw macadamia nuts and a few walnuts
Lunch: 5-6 spicy, large green and black olives, spinach salad with sunflower seeds and spinach-almond pesto
Snack: almonds, pumpkin seeds, spinach salad, vinegar and oil dressing, corn, zucchini and yellow squash
Dinner: raw peas and carrot and garlic salad with olive oil
Snack: 0

Day 6 clogging
Breakfast: 1/2 red grapefruit
Snack: 0
Lunch: My Big Basic Salad Bowl with avocado and spinach-almond pesto
Snack: 0
Dinner: avocado, red pepper, grated carrot and miso dressing
Snack: 2 nut-seed balls

Day 7 yoga
Breakfast: Power Smoothie
Snack: herb tea, 2 ABC cookies
Lunch: 1 apple, 1 tangerine, a handful of raw nuts
Snack: a few bites of Cauliflower Mash with flax oil
Dinner: 2-3 green olives
Snack: 0

Week 8
Day 1 step aerobics, weights
Breakfast: Power Smoothie
Snack: 0
Lunch: Super Sushi Roll with grated carrots, Hearty Party Dip, raw asparagus, sprouts, avocado and miso dressing
Snack: 0
Dinner: 1 grapefruit

Day 2 yoga
Breakfast: Power Smoothie
Snack: herbal tea
Lunch: olives, Savory Herb Bread with mashed avocado
Snack: Sprouted Wheat, Raisin, Cinnamon Bread with nut butter
Dinner: herbal tea, a few raw seeds and raisins, dried figs
Snack: 0

Day 3 step aerobics, weights
Breakfast: 0
Snack: 1 apple
Lunch: My Big Basic Salad Bowl, small size, 1 Super Sushi Roll
Snack: Oregon Hummus with raw carrots and jicama and broccoli
Dinner: celery stalks with nut butter, avocado slices, tomato slices
Snack: tea, Cinn-fully Delicious Yogurt

Day 4 clogging
Breakfast: Power Smoothie
Snack: 2-3 pecan-stuffed dates
Lunch: 1/2 avocado and cucumber slices, mini-carrots
Snack: cucumber slices, Oregon Hummus, marinated chickpeas, carrots
Dinner: 1 apple, raw nuts
Snack: 2 Fudgies

Day 5 yoga
Breakfast: 2 kiwi fruit, 4 strawberries, 1/2 banana, sliced into a salad with nutmeg
Snack: grape juice
Lunch: carrots, broccoli, olives, snap peas, cherry tomatoes on platter with sprouts and greens and dressing
Snack: 2 Fudgies
Dinner: Power Smoothie

Day 6 walk, yoga
Breakfast: ginger, cayenne, maple syrup tea
Snack: more tea
Lunch: a little avocado and miso dressing spread on Savory Herb Bread
Snack: 3 roll-ups using large lettuce leaves - filling was Golden Mayo, grated carrot and red cabbage, cucumbers, avocado and red pepper
Dinner: Sprouted Wheat, Raisin, Cinnamon Bread with nut butter and sliced bananas
Snack: Power Smoothie

Day 7 walk
Breakfast: grape juice
Snack: Power Smoothie
Lunch: My Big Basic Salad Bowl
Snack: 1/2 avocado, cucumber slices, Spicy Jicama 'Stix' with lime juice and onion powder
Dinner: almonds, olives, walnuts
Snack: 1 tangerine

Week 9
Day 1 yoga
Breakfast: 1 kiwi
Snack: Power Smoothie with 2 kale leaves
Lunch: My Big Basic Salad Bowl
Snack: 0
Dinner: 1 grapefruit

Day 2 no exercise
Breakfast: 1 tangelo
Snack: herb tea
Lunch: Spicy Jicama 'Stix', My Big Basic Salad Bowl with Mi Miso Dressing
Snack: 1/2 banana
Dinner: Earthshaking Shake
Snack: 0

Day 3 yoga
Breakfast: Power Shake (Berry Berry Blue - cashew milk with vanilla, protein powder, frozen banana chunks and 1/2 cup blueberries)
Snack: 0
Lunch: red Swiss chard salad with yellow squash, zucchini, red onion, cucumber, spinach, corn, grated raw beets, carrots, vinegar and oil and herb dressing
Snack: 0
Dinner: fruit salad - with oranges, strawberries, banana, kiwi
Snack: 0

Day 4 yoga, walk
Breakfast: Detox tea
Snack: 1 orange
Lunch: My Big Basic Salad Bowl, Veggie-Nut Patty, Sunrise Sauce, Broccoli-in-Bed, Spicy Jicama 'Stix', 2 Marbles
Snack: 0
Dinner: 0
Snack: 2 Marbles

Day 5 clogging
Breakfast: 1/2 banana, 1 t. raw tahini
Snack: 1 apple, 1 store-bought raw cookie
Lunch: My Big Basic Salad Bowl
Snack: a few nuts, some avocado
Dinner: rest of My Big Basic Salad Bowl
Snack: red grapefruit

Day 6 walk
Breakfast: 1 banana dipped in almond butter
Snack: 0
Lunch: Power Smoothie
Snack: 1/2 avocado with dressing
Dinner: My Big Basic Salad Bowl
Snack: 1 cherimoya - yummy

Day 7 walk, yoga
Breakfast: tea
Snack: some nuts
Lunch: 2 ugli fruit, several bites of durian, some hijiki, grated carrot, gobo salad with rice vinegar
Snack: 3 Fudgies and herb tea, more hijiki, grated carrot, gobo salad and some avocado
Dinner: 1 ugli fruit
Snack: 1 Fudgie Ball

Week 10
Day 1 walk
Breakfast: Power Smoothie
Snack: herb tea
Lunch: My Big Basic Salad Bowl with rest of hijiki salad, sprouts, avocado, snap peas, broccoli, tomatoes, etc.
Snack: 2 Fudgie Balls, 1 date
Dinner: 1 bowl fruit salad (1/2 banana, 1 mango, 1 kiwi, 3-4 strawberries)
Snack: 1 cara cara orange

Day 2 walk
Breakfast: 1 apple, 1 banana
Snack: Warm Carob 'Mocha-Chai' tea - I made with Sweet & Spicy tea, almond milk, carob powder, maple syrup
Lunch: My Big Basic Salad Bowl
Snack: orange and pineapple juice with ice cubes, blended - like an Icee, rest of My Big Basic Salad Bowl
Dinner: Fruit Salad (1 pear, 3 strawberries, 1/2 cara cara orange, 1 kiwi and Five Spice Powder)
Snack: 2 Fudgie Balls

Day 3 clogging
Breakfast: 1 honey tangerine
Snack: 0
Lunch: 1 apple, several mini-carrots, 1 pink grapefruit
Snack: 3 cara cara oranges, 1 pink grapefruit, 1 tray ice-blended in blender
Dinner: 1/2 avocado with Veg-It
Snack: 1/2 avocado with spring greens, miner's lettuce, broccoli shreds, red pepper and cucumber
Snack: 2 Fudgie Balls

Day 4 step aerobics
Breakfast: 1 kiwi, 1 apple
Snack: 0
Lunch: Power Shake (Berry Berry Blue - almond milk with blueberries, frozen bananas, protein powder and 1 t. nutritional yeast)
Snack: 1/2 avocado with Veg-It
Dinner: 1 grapefruit, 3 Fudgie Balls
Snack: 1 tangerine

Day 5 step aerobics, weights
Breakfast: 1 green pear, Power Shake (Berry Berry Blue with almond milk, frozen bananas and blueberries)
Snack: strawberries, apple slices
Lunch: My Big Basic Salad Bowl with miner's lettuce, sprouts, avocado, red pepper, cucumbers, shredded broccoli and carrots, sunflower seeds, tahini dressing
Snack: 3 Fudgie Balls, small helping Cauliflower Mash with flax seed oil, 3 strawberries, 1 organic banana
Dinner: Power Smoothie with red Swiss chard leaves, frozen strawberries
Snack: dried figs, dried, juicy plums (no sulfur dioxide), 4 Medjool dates

Day 6 clogging
Breakfast: 1 organic banana
Snack: fresh strawberries, 1 orange
Lunch: Power Shake (with almond milk, strawberries, orange juice, nutritional yeast, protein powder, miner's lettuce, flax seed)
Snack: 1/2 avocado, 3 bites Cauliflower Mash, a few cashews
Dinner: 1 small tangerine, My Big Basic Salad Bowl with sprouts and miner's lettuce, red leaf lettuce, butter lettuce, shredded broccoli, red pepper, cucumbers, fresh, black olive dressing and green salsa
Snack: 2 Medjool dates, 4 dried, moist plums, 3 dried figs

Day 7 yoga
Breakfast: carob-date-banana-almond milk shake
Snack: fresh pineapple slices, organic red grapes
Lunch: 1 Super Sushi Roll lined with lettuces, sprouts, miner's lettuce, red pepper, cucumbers, Roma tomatoes, avocado, olive dressing and avocado, lots of Lani's Tomatillo Salsa Rocks
Snack: 1/2 organic banana, 2 strawberries, 1 apple, sliced, some nuts
Dinner: small salad with greens, miner's lettuce, avocado, and tomatoes and olive oil and lemon juice dressing
Snack: 2 dried figs, 3-4 dried, juicy plums, 3 Marbles

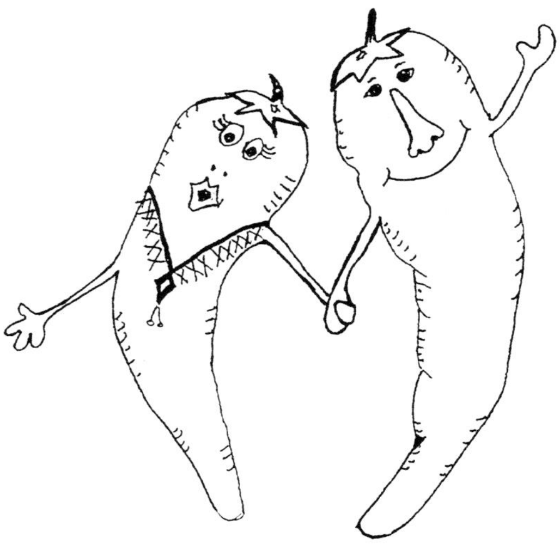

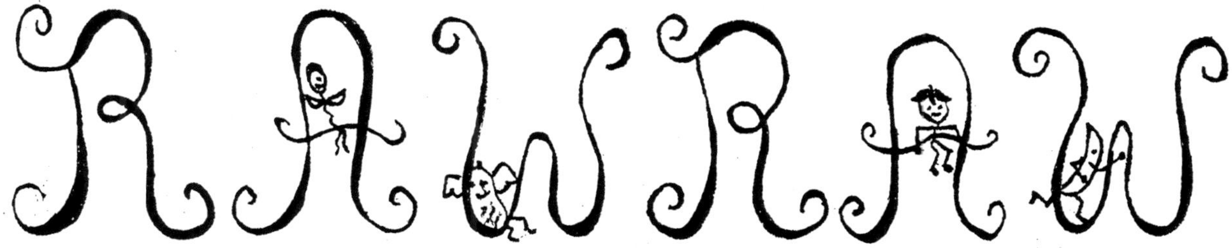

CHAPTER XI
WHAT'S NEXT?
(AFTER TEN WEEKS AND A SIGNIFICANT WEIGHT LOSS)

My Total Weight Loss for the First 10 Weeks was twenty-five pounds. I treated myself at the end of each week. Sometimes it was an article of clothing, especially when I had to give away my old larger sized jeans. Other times it was a new CD or book or some beads to make a pretty bracelet or necklace.

Halfway through the Live Food Eating Plan I traveled to Portland to be with my daughter. I was wondering how I would make it through my first time away from home. Fortunately I brought salad ingredients with me and some of the ingredients for my Power Smoothie. I also bought fresh fruit while I was there and a fresh spinach pesto. The week-end turned out to be successful. For the first time I wasn't tempted by her various candy dishes (always full) or her containers of cookies and other crunchy snacks. By five weeks, I felt in control and so happy I was losing weight and eating only highly nutritious food that I didn't want to put anything 'dead' in my body.

One day my daughter and I went shopping. I wanted new tops to replace some of my 'fat' tops. We were in the dressing room trying on tops. Much to my delight, my daughter had to take a few items back and return with smaller sizes. That felt really great, as usually the opposite is true. I felt like I had another successful turning point on this path toward wellness and fitness.

Exercise helped me raise my metabolism. Notice how I varied my exercise routine, from day to day. If you like to walk and have a friend to walk with 3 or 4 times a week, or headphones to listen to a tape or music, then by all means, stick with the same exercise. Having a few weights, 1 lb., 5 lb., 8 lb. lying around the house, makes it easy to do some weight lifting while you are watching television or listening to music. If you don't belong to a gym or health club, invest in a couple of video exercise tapes. Some of my favorites are a 20 minute yoga routine to do before bedtime (very relaxing), a dance aerobics tape and a step aerobics tape. I also have tried Tae Bo (like kick-boxing) and belly-dancing tapes.

Whatever gets you to move, including parking farther away from where you are going, walking up the stairs instead of the elevator and doing morning stretches, will increase your metabolism and energy. If you like to swim or bicycle, by all means find a way to do so, indoors or outside. I have scootered with my grand-kids and inline skated along our community bike path. It's all invigorating and will change your attitude about aging. You will feel more youthful just by moving and be even more inspired to stick with this eating plan.

Diary at End of Ten Weeks

Ten weeks ago I set out to re-create my body and improve my health. Losing weight was the immediate objective, since I had been literally unable to lose weight in the past several years, no matter what "diet" I tried.

Now, ten weeks later, I am 25 pounds lighter, having lost 2 pounds a week steadily after dropping an initial 5 pounds of bloat and water the first week. I not only have gone from size Large and Extra-Large in my tops to size Petite Small, and decreased from size 10-12 to 6-8 in my pants size, but I feel healthier than I ever have.

The so-called "normal" aches and pains, stiffness, etc. that we have come to tolerate as we get older have disappeared. A little eczema by my right ear has disappeared. My blood pressure has gone from borderline high to normal. The swelling in my ankles at the end of the day, which had occurred ever since last summer when I almost got heat stroke building an outdoor labyrinth in 105 degree heat, disappeared. My skin is clear and smooth. Wrinkles still there but seem to be diminished. There is no puffiness under my eyes.

My mind is clearer, calmer and more alert. I require less sleep and awaken early and ready to rise. I have higher energy and stamina than ever before.

My spirit is at peace. I see this world through different eyes; I feel it differently. There is clarity in my sense of purpose. Through my intuition and not through what I read, I have listened to my body and let it guide me.

After the first few weeks I discontinued my main vitamins, calcium, vitamin C and vitamin E. A week or so later I stopped the B complex vitamins. The only artificial man-made supplements I take are nutritional yeast (approx. 1 T.), 2-3 times a week in my Power Smoothie, and the Super Green, soy-based protein powder I also add to the same fruit or nut-milk based smoothie or shake.

My body, I am confident, is more alive and detoxified on the inside. The cells are less congested and more able to perform the marvelous functions they were intended to do.

I exercise with joy, something I look forward to.

I feel transformed, cell by cell, into a new person-inside and outside. I will continue to lose weight naturally by eating living foods only, because every fruit, vegetable, nut, seed or sprout is packed with the raw materials my body needs for growth, maintenance or repair and rejuvenation.

The remaining pounds of fat will burn off until the wisdom of my body decides there is no more excess fat to get rid of. The live enzymes continue to burn fat in my body.

Whereas my former self would have said, "I want to lose 15 more pounds," my new self listens to my body and allows it to decide how much more weight, in the form of fat, will go.

I have received insights I never had before. It is as though a light bulb went on and I had a few "aha" moments, where I could see everything clearly, all at once. Reading books on raw foods by raw-foodists, some of whom were medical doctors, most of whom have written about increased health benefits they personally experienced as well as testimonials from their fellow raw food enthusiasts has certainly enhanced my beliefs. But there is absolutely nothing like experiencing increased health. Knowing what I now know, and feeling what I now feel, there is no going back.

It's almost the same as when I first became a vegetarian. After reading "Diet for a Small Planet," by Frances Moore Lappe', I knew too much--about what happens ecologically, environmentally, ethically and healthwise when we eat meat, that I couldn't consciously ever eat meat again. Fish left my dinner table a bit later, as did dairy products and eggs.

I would like to recommend "Mad Cowboy," a book I just finished reading. It was written by Howard F. Lyman, the ex-cattle rancher who was on Oprah's show a few years ago. It was because of what he said that got Oprah in trouble with the Meat Industry when she stated she'd never eat a burger again. Fortunately, she won her suit. The book is full of facts and is much more important to the health and survival of our planet than anything else I have read. Like Rachael Carson's 'Silent Spring' which warned us, among other things, about the dangers of pesticides in our crops.

Howard, as a former high tech rancher himself, warns us of how close we are to total soil depletion, water pollution and depletion and air pollution, due to the dangerous practices of modern day cattle and dairy farming techniques. He tells it like it is and he has the inside track. It's so much more about our planet and what is happening all around the globe, including the millions of acres disappearing from our rain forests to satisfy the primarily American love affair with hamburgers.

We are losing our oxygen, our topsoil, our viable lands due to the almighty cow. It's also about the pesticides, hormones and antibiotics in your meat, Mad Cow disease or cannibalism in their feed. It's time we all woke up and saw the absurdity of feeding the cattle our grains, in fact, 20 pounds of grain for every resulting pound of hamburger. Isn't that getting protein second-hand? A waste of land and seed? Well, you decide. The 11 Western states use 70% of their water for cattle raising. Go to your library, check out the book and read the first 50 pages, and then read more, if you dare. Or read the Chapter on Bovine Planet and see if you can read more. Discuss it with your friends. Buy the book and pass it on to others. We all, collectively must do something. We must change our dependence on meat and dairy. We have been misled by the two most powerful, government-connected forces in our country. The third one, very connected to both, plus the government is Monsanto Chemical Company. Read and see what each one's agenda is--not your health, not the truth about the safety of what they peddle, but pure greed at the expense of those of us in blissful ignorance. We must wake up before it is too late.

I write this because I want to both warn you and encourage you. Regarding the eating plan, be prepared to feel better than ever after 10 weeks. You will lose weight. Then be prepared that it might change your life forever.

I tell you truly, the last 5 weeks and continuing to this very moment, as I write these words, I simplify more and more, eating fresh fruit alone, or sometimes mixed with a few other fruits. I make a large salad with lots of greens, juicy vegetables, such as tomatoes, cucumbers and red pepper, with a few others for variety and a sprinkling of nuts. Always, avocado tops my salad and a homemade dressing adorns it. For dinner I often enjoy a piece of fruit. I sprout sometimes, but keep it simple. The variety of fruits, vegetables, seeds, nuts and sprouts, makes it easy to vary my own salads. It is never boring. Look how many varieties of apples there are to try. More and more oranges, grapefruits, tangerines and ugli fruit is available to enjoy.

I heard that one raw food expert states a very wise and practical way to look at eating raw foods. He has a 5-5-5 rule. Don't make any meal that has over 5 ingredients in it, costs more than $5.00 or takes more than 5 minutes to prepare. I like that. Too many fruits mixed together or too many vegetables in a salad might be harder to digest and may not follow standard food-combining rules.

So far I have never been too hungry, nor too full, and I did not have any digestive difficulties the entire 10 weeks. Normally, in that span of time, I would either have overeaten and the food would cause either gas or make me uncomfortable, or I would have eaten too many combinations, also causing gas and bloating. I also used to eat too late at night and the food would sit there all night, not moving or being digested. Very uncomfortable. None of this has happened to me on the live foods eating plan. I like going to bed with very little in my stomach. I lay on my back and my stomach feels flat and empty. This contributes to a good night's sleep. And my restless leg syndrome has all but disappeared.

I make simple salad dressings, some nut milks and seed cheeses. I dehydrate ripe fruit or veggies for chips or chews. Life is much simpler; I only shop the produce aisle and never have to make decisions about what to buy. I never read labels anymore because my food is packed in its own edible container-the skin. There are no labels to read about nutritional content.

I try to buy organic and fresh; however, even commercially grown fruits and vegetables eaten raw are healthier than cooked organic, processed foods.

Let's review *my* plan. On New Year's Day, I made a conscious decision to take control of my eating and lose weight. I was sick of having no waistline, a protruding stomach, big upper arms, etc. I never wore anything tucked in, nor sleeveless tops. I decided to ignore my taste buds. How ridiculous to let a few taste buds on your tongue dictate, simply by taste, what one shovels into one's mouth.

I would ignore or divert any psychological addictions such as a run to the nearest coffee shop to get a mocha, or eating when I'm bored or out of habit for a mid-afternoon snack, usually something sweet. I decided to give no power to any thought, nor take any action when I experienced a physical craving. What I previously followed through on when I had a physical craving I now channel into eating a piece of fruit, a handful of nuts or a smoothie, giving no energy or "thought" to what my body was addicted to, i.e. chocolate, mochas, candy, starches. It became a non-issue.

My decision to eat raw occluded any candy, chocolate or coffee. I prepared a few sweets out of carob, raw maple syrup and nuts or nut butters to substitute for days I felt out of control. They were tasty, but after 4 or 5 days I lost my cravings for sweets. Somehow the sweet taste of fruits and the greens, rich in vitamins and minerals, establish a balance in blood sugar levels and the craving for sweets disappears. The sweet cravings gave up on me. I can consciously eat and enjoy one or two sweet carob nut balls and not crave eating the entire "batch."

Eating For a Lifetime of Energy and Good Health

Now that you are ____ pounds lighter and feeling great in your new clothes, you'll want to maintain that weight loss. Your weight-loss should stabilize at the best weight for you. Listen to your body. Listen to your new body, because you have rid yourself of many of the toxins and 'sludge' of your previous habits that prevented you from losing weight. When your cells are receiving nothing but nutrient-dense foods, they will know when the extra fat is gone.

Studies have shown that nutrient-rich foods can be eaten with minimal calories and you will be healthy and possibly live longer. So, appreciate the new health your body radiates.

Try to remember or review your daily food journal to see what your triggers were. Think about any little health problems that have minimized or disappeared, even little things, like your hair shines more, your skin is clearer, your bowel movements regular without the aid of laxatives. Your skin might be balanced - neither too dry, nor too oily. When you get out of bed your joints aren't stiff. You have more stamina, require less sleep and awake fully alert, both morning and early evening. Write them down and ask yourself, isn't this the result of my new body, due to my new way of eating and moving?

1. After 10 weeks, re-evaluate and decide what cooked foods you might want to gradually add to your new lifetime eating plan. Remember, you can continue on this program for life. Adding a small amount of cooked foods would really be for convenience, because you're cooking for your family or because you really miss certain foods and haven't found a satisfactory substitute. If you really miss sour dough bread, for instance, and don't find the sprouted, dehydrated breads satisfactory, then allow yourself to have some once in awhile along with your family. Just don't get hooked on previous habits, such as eating several slices slathered with butter along with pasta - both highly refined carbohydrate foods. Be sensible, but splurge every now and then.

However, if you went totally, 100% raw for 10 weeks, then you must be very careful when re-introducing cooked foods. From what I've read, anyone who has thought they could have a cooked meal, usually gets a toxic reaction from their body. Just as one usually comes off a fast with juices, then a few steamed vegetables, one needs to treat cooked foods in the same manner, something to re-introduce into one's diet, very slowly, in small amounts. Pay attention to your body and notice how it feels, before, during and after your first cooked food after eating entirely raw for so many weeks.

2. Decide to eat 1 totally raw meal a day, or 2 totally raw meals a week. You might choose to eat 5 totally raw meals a week. This way, you could try a totally living foods breakfast one day, a living foods lunch another day, an uncooked dinner another, alternating throughout the week. Alternatively, you could add a few raw items to every meal you eat. That's quite easy. Eat fresh fruit in the morning, a salad for lunch and dinner, raw nuts or fruit for snacks.

3. Look over the menus and recipes and decide to try a few. Incorporate them into your current eating plan as you eliminate or reduce your intake of highly refined carbohydrates (sugars, starches i.e. white flour, breads, crackers) and high fat junk foods, i.e. bacon, hamburger, French fries, and potato chips. You might decide to incorporate more salads and fresh fruits into your daily eating plan, while continuing to eat something cooked at each meal. You could buy raw nuts rather than roasted, which are much more nutritious. You could try to sprout some seeds to add more live foods to your salads. This might help you eliminate some processed, packaged food and substitute with food from the produce section of your super market.

4. Important! If you went totally raw for 5 weeks or even 10, and now want to add some cooked foods back into your diet, i.e. a baked potato, steamed rice, etc., be very careful to add something very slowly and in a very small quantity. Your body isn't used to cooked food, so don't go eat a large bowl of rice or a big baked potato with butter. You might begin with 1/4 cup of steamed rice, or 1/4 of a baked potato with flax oil. Always have a green salad with anything cooked. Be careful.

However you choose, reduce the junk food, caffeine, refined starches and sugars. Add more salads, raw vegetables and fruit to your meals, and you will continue to lose or maintain that weight.

Happy Eating!

And now I leave you with two thoughts, one from my favorite place, Hawaii (I lived there as a teen-ager) and one from the birthplace of my grandparents:

See everything, feel everything, think everything, and always try to be in Io, Kala, Ke Aloha (Truth, Light and Love).

Swedish Proverb:

Fear less, hope more; eat less, chew more
Whine less, breathe more; talk less, say more
Hate less, love more; and all good things are yours.

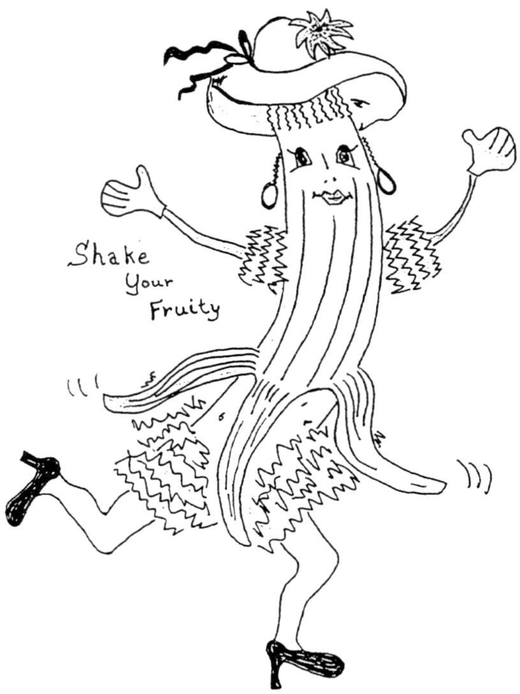

RAW FOOD WEBSITES

www.1stchoicenutritionals.com - First Choice Nutritionals
www.annwigmore.org - Ann Wigmore Institute
www.cherylstoycoff.com - Cheryl's Pages
www.davidwolfe.com - David Wolfe
www.diamondorganics.com - Diamond Organics
www.eatveg.com - Eat Veg!
www.ecoforest.org - Raw Food Eco-village Project
www.eco-organics.com - Eco-Organics
www.fresh-network.com - Fresh Network
www.fresh-network.com - The FRESH Network
www.gardenofhealth.com - Garden of Health
www.HealthCreation.net
www.healthforce.net - HealthForce Nutritionals
www.healthfullivingintl.com - Healthful Living International
www.highvibe.com - High Vibe Health & Healing
www.justeatanapple.com - Just Eat an Apple Magazine
www.livingnutrition.com - Living Nutrition Magazine
www.purejoylivingfoods.com - Pure Joy Living Foods
www.rawfamily.com - Raw Family
www.rawfood.com - Nature's First Law
www.rawfoodchef.com - Living Light Culinary Arts Institute
www.rawfoodliving.com - Raw Food Living
www.rawfoodnews.com - Raw Foods News
www.rawfoods.com - Living-Foods Community
www.rawgourmet.com - The Raw Gourmet
www.rawhealth.net - Raw Health
www.rawheaven.com - Raw Heaven
www.rawlife.com - Raw Life
www.rawolution.com - Rawolution
www.rawvegan.com - Raw Vegan International
www.shazzie.com - Shazzie
www.sunfood.net - The Sunfood Cuisine
www.thelivingtemple.com - The Living Temple
www.TheRawWorld.com - Raw Life
www.treeoflife.com - Tree of Life Rejuvenation Center
www.vibrantliving.com - Institute for Vibrant Living
www.vitalities.org - Vitalities Incorporated

RECOMMENDED READING

Boutenko, Victoria, Igor, Sergei and Valya. *Raw Family.* Ashland, Oregon: Raw Family Publishing, 2000.

Boutenko, Sergei and Valya. *Eating Without Heating.* Ashland, Oregon: Raw Family Publishing, 2002.

Boutenko, Victoria. *12 Steps to Raw Foods.* Ashland, Oregon: Raw Family Publishing, 2002.

Cousens, Gabriel, M.D. *Conscious Eating.* Berkeley, California: North Atlantic Books, 2000.

Howell, Dr. Edward. *Enzyme Nutrition-The Food Enzyme Concept.* Wayne, New Jersey: Avery Publishing Group, 1985.

Juliano. *Raw-The UNcook Book.* New York, NY: Regan Books, 1999.

Lyman, Howard. *Mad Cowboy.* New York, NY: Touchstone, 1998.

Meyerowitz, Steve. *Sprouts-The Miracle Food.* Great Barrington, Massachusetts: The Sprout House, Inc., 1983 (Seventh Printing, 1997).

Miller, Susie and Karen Knowles. *feel-good food.* London, England: The Women's Press Ltd., 2000.

Patenaude, Frederic. *Sunfood Cuisine.* San Diego, California: Genesis 1:29 Publishing, 2001.

Rhio. *Hooked on Raw.* New York, NY: Beso Entertainment, 2000.

Shannon, Nomi. *The Raw Gourmet.* Burnaby, BC: Alive Books, 1999.

Wigmore, Andd, D.D., N.D. *Why You Do Not Need to Grow Old.* USA: Ann Wigmore, 1985.

Wolfe, David. *The Sunfood Diet Success System.* San Diego, California: Maui Brothers Publishing, 2001.

Magazine: "Just Eat an Apple". Editor: Frederic Patenaude. Published by Raw Vegan Publishing Co., Montreal, Quebec, Canada.

ABOUT THE AUTHOR

Lani Rossetta is an occupational therapist, former school teacher, Reiki master and yoga instructor. She has worked with children all her life, as her publications reflect.

Lil' Smarty - a reading-readiness board game.
We Love Your Body - a natural foods nutrition and cook book for kids and adults.
Granny Gecko Stories - a series of five environment-friendly, fantasy, children's stories.
How to Keep Your Angel Fit - a children's story about keeping one's angel fit.
Labyrinth Llama - a llama doll pattern.
Don't Prick Me, You Little Stick - a humorous needle book and carrying case.
Frieda Frõga - a frog doll pattern with wired arms and legs to put in any of the yoga postures. Comes with instructions to sew as well as making her own lily pad to do the exercises on.
Labyrinths for Kids - A book full of ideas for using labyrinths as a tool for increasing fine motor, gross motor and visual perceptual skills in kids in the classroom.
Frieda Frõga Loves to Yoga - The first Frõga Yoga book for kids.
Freddie Frõga Loves to Yoga, II - The second Frõga Yoga book for kids.
Nikki & Little Lily Frõga Love to Yoga, III - The third Frõga Yoga book for kids.
Nikki, Lily Frõga & Friends Create Nutritious & Tasty Bug Treats - Sixteen delicious recipes with photos that Nikki, Lily & Friends teach kids to create in their kitchen in an easy-to-read book. For 5-11 year-old children.
Let's Have a Labyrinth Party - a handbook with hundreds of ideas for celebrations on, in and around a labyrinth. Food, decorations, games, patterns and more. 53 pages of photos, local labyrinths in and around Southern Oregon and Northern California.
Lose Weight With Live Foods! A 10 week plan to lose fat and gain health and fitness - a book full of recipes for preparing raw, living foods; includes a 10 week plan for dropping the excess fat through eating live foods. Lots of tips, personal stories, information on the benefits of eating raw.

In her spare time Lani enjoys yoga, hiking, bicycling, reading, knitting socks, making dolls, traveling, metaphysics, teaching labyrinth workshops, teaching raw food preparation classes and playing with the grandkids. She is a relatively new raw food enthusiast.

Please write the author if you have any questions or wish to locate or order any of her books or patterns. Some are sold at www.amazon.com while others can be ordered at the following address:

Lani Rossetta - 5205 Dobrot Way, Central Point, OR 97502
Phone: 541-664-4531 email: leihuna@cdsnet.net
Website: www.home.internetcds.com/~leihuna

PHOTOS

BEFORE 10 WEEK EATING PLAN

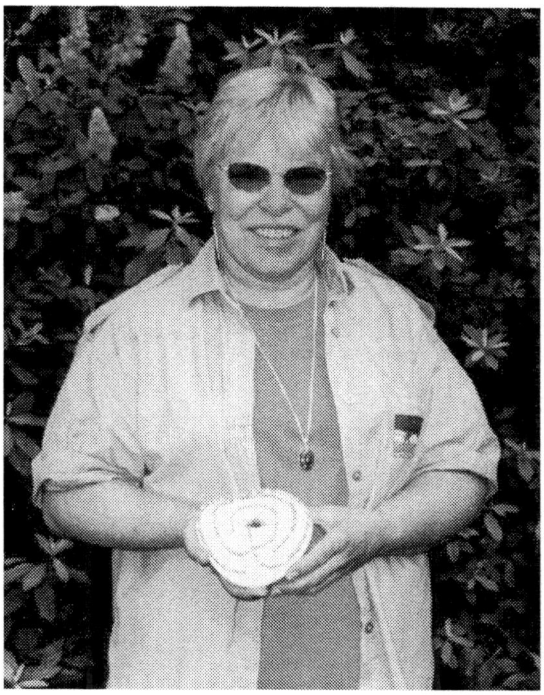

AFTER 10 WEEKS OF LIVE FOODS

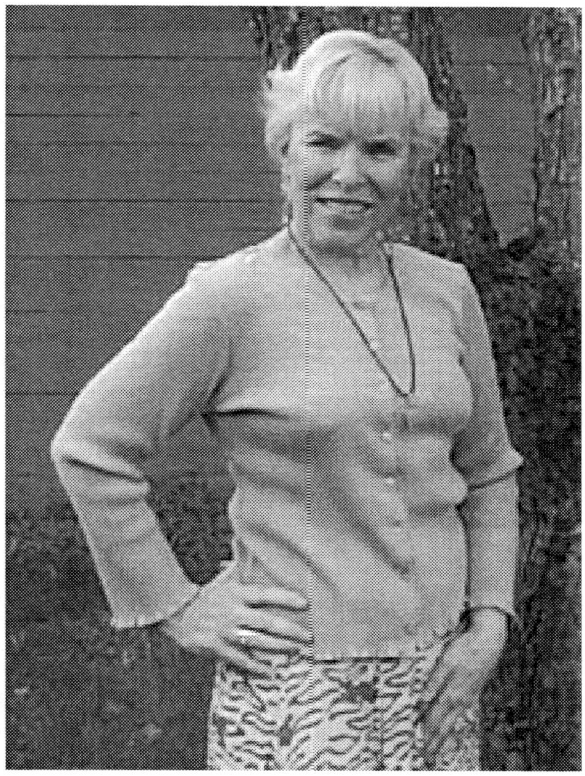

NOTES

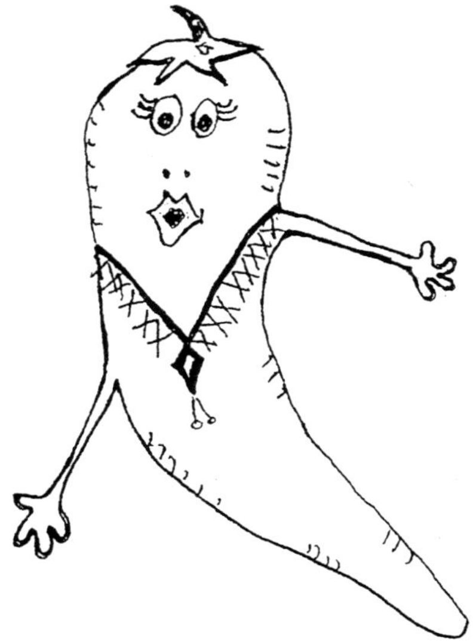

RECIPE INDEX

Drink to Your Health:

Juices 35

Liquid Sunshine
Rainbow Blend
Apple-Ginger Zinger
Salute to the Sun
Green Spiral
Liver Detoxifying Drink
Jubilation Celebration
Aloha Nui
Vitamin Energizer
V-6 Wake Up
Pineapple Plus Energy Drinks
Herbal Teas
Healthy Soda Pop
Rejuvelac

Smoothies 40

Super Smoothies
Carob-Date
Pineapple Berry
Beta Blue Smoothie
Mellow Yellow
Strawberry Smoothie
Power Smoothie-Power Shake
Peach Smoothie
Sunny Apple Flax Seed Smoothie
La Luna Freeze

Shakes 45

Super Milk Shakes
Got a Date with a Fig Shake
Carob-Banana Shake
Thick and Fruity
Janet's Bone Builder Shake
Earthshaking Shake
Almond-Cinnamon Mixture

Nut and Seed Milks 47

Generic Nut Milk
Almond Milk for One or Two People
A Quart of Almond Milk
Sesame Seed Milk
Sweet Cashew-Date Milk
Warm Carob Cocoa
Warm Carob 'Mocha-Chai'

Lively Sprouts:

Growing Sprouts 55

Sunflower Seed Sprouts
Wheat Sprouts
Mixed Sprouts
Sprout Combos
Mung Sprouts
Wheatgrass
Buckwheat or Sunflower Lettuce
Mini-Lesson on Soaking Nuts & Seeds
Captain Buckwheat Crunch
Blanching Almonds
Twelve Ways to Eat Your Sprouts!

Breads, Crackers, Cereals 60

Breads 60

Sprouted Wheat, Raisin, Cinnamon Bread
Savory Herb Bread
Chapatis

Crackers 61

Flax Crackers
Crisp Buckwheat Frisbees

Cereals 62

Whole Grain Cereal
Muesli
Grape Nutty Cereal
Blueberry Breakfast

Snacks:

Sweet Snacks 65

South of the Border Bananas
Funny Faces
Fresh Applesauce with Cinnamon
Layered Parfait Dessert
Fruit Kebobs

Spicy Snacks 66

Spicy Captain Buckwheat Crunch
Crisp Buckwheat Frisbees
Spicy Jicama 'Stix'
Mushroom Caps
Wholly Guacamole
Easy 'Cup' Snacks
Chips Ahoy!
More Chips for Dips

Frozen Snacks 70

Jawbreakers
Carob-Banana Pops
Carob Sauce
Snow Cones
Popsicles

On-the-Go Snacks 71

Gummy Bugs
Pick-Me-Ups
Stuffed Snacks
Cup O' Crunch
Banana Burrito!
Tooty Fruity Burrito!
Stuffed Apple Lunch
Live Foods Trail Mix
Hiking Energy Trail Balls
Sprouts, Raisins and Dates
Dried Fruit Roll-ups
Barb's Sweet Sugar Plums

Food Processor Magic:

Sauces 75

Seed Sauce
Sunrise Sauce
Pecan Sauce
Mushroom Sauce
'Hot Tamale' Sauce
Pizza Sauce
Spinach Pesto
Basil Pesto
Sprouted Sunflower Seed Sauce
Fruity Seed Sauce

Dips-Spreads 79

Hearty Party Dip
Green, Creamy Dip
Oregon Hummus
Cauliflower Mash
Party Pate'
Sprouted Sunflower Seed Dip

Butters 82

Nut and Seed Butters
Nut Butter With . . .
Tahini Spread
Tahini Topping
Peach Lover's Delight
Monkey Mash
'Cheese, Sprouts, and Nut Butter
Avocado Butter
'We Love Your Body' Guacamole
Green Goddess Better Butter

Salsas 85

Pineapple Salsa
WLYB Salsa
Cheryl's Tropical Salsa
Green Salsa Challenge
High C Salsa